INTRODUCTION TO HEALTH EDUCATION describes the practice of health education, emphasizing the present and future role of the health educator as an agent of behavioral change. It presents a systematic model of educational change that can be used to create realistic change strategies in individuals and in a variety of settings. Included are case studies and an overview of the future directions of health education.

Please turn to the back of the book for other Mayfield titles of interest to health educators.

INTRODUCTION

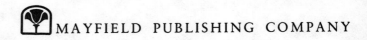

MAYFIELD PUBLISHING COMPANY

TO
HEALTH
EDUCATION

IRA J. BATES

ALVIN E. WINDER
University of Massachusetts, Amherst

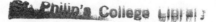

Library of Congress Catalog Card Number: 83-061536
International Standard Book Number: 0-87484-586-6

Manufactured in the United States of America
Mayfield Publishing Company
285 Hamilton Avenue
Palo Alto, California 94301

Sponsoring editor: C. Lansing Hays
Manuscript editor: Joy Dickinson
Managing editor: Pat Herbst
Art director: Nancy Sears
Illustrator: Pat Rogondino
Production manager: Cathy Willkie
Compositor: Auto-Graphics
Printer and binder: Bookcrafters

Credits

Pages 64, 65, 66 Selections reprinted from *Change: Principles of Problem Formation and Problem Resolution*, by Paul Watzlawick, John Weakland, and Richard Fisch, by permission of W. W. Norton & Company, Inc. Copyright © 1974 by W. W. Norton & Company, Inc.

Pages 97, 116 Reprinted from R. M. Henig, "East Kentucky's Answer: A Model for the Future," pp. 24–27. Copyright © June 1976 by *The New Physician*.

Pages 129, 136 Reprinted from *Health and Health Care Policies in Perspective* by A. R. Somers and H. M. Somers by permission of Aspen Systems Corporation, © 1976.

Pages 163–70 Reprinted from Charlotte N. Spiegel and Francis C. Lindaman, "Children Can't Fly: A Program to Prevent Childhood Morbidity and Mortality from Window Falls," pp. 1143–1146. Copyright © 1977 by the American Public Health Association.

Page 170–74 Reprinted from Leslie Fisher, Virginia Goddard Harris, John VanBuren, John Quinn, and Alison DeMaio, "Assessment of a Pilot Child Playground Injury Prevention Project in New York State," pp. 1000–1002. Copyright © 1980 by the American Public Health Association.

Page 174–83 Reprinted from R. A. Dersheivitz and J. W. Williamson, "Prevention of Childhood Household Injuries: A Controlled Clinical Trial," pp. 1148–1153. Copyright © 1977 by the American Public Health Association.

Page 220 Figure 10.1 reprinted from Alan C. Henderson, John M. Wollfe, Peter A. Cortese, and Deborah V. McIntosh, "The Future of the Health Education Profession: Implications for Preparation and Practice," *Public Health Reports*, November–December 1981, Vol. 96, No. 6, p. 558. Copyright © 1981 by *Public Health Reports*.

Contents

Chapter 5
Understanding Health Education Practice   92

Chapter 6
Health Education Programs: Settings for Practice   107

Preface

This book brings together, in a single conceptual framework, the diverse practice that currently defines the field of health education. We believe that health education is a field whose practice is crucial to the implementation of any effective program of prevention; we hope to encourage and nurture a similar understanding in students. Our challenge has been to provide a health education text that is both acceptable and readable at the undergraduate and beginning graduate levels.

In writing this book, we had four major goals. First, we wanted to develop a theoretical model of educational change for the health field. The model we have conceived clarifies four types of change, each type of which requires a unique strategy for change and suggests a guide for appropriate level of health education practice. Second, we hoped to suggest a theoretical model as a guide for the specific practice of health education change. In doing so, we have provided a way to define a health setting, predict the outcome of an effective health education strategy, and assess the skills needed to obtain that outcome. Third, we intended to illustrate the diagnostic use of our change model; thus, we have used a number of case studies of health problems relevant to health education to illustrate our method of diagnosis. And fourth, we determined to illustrate the use of our practice model in a series of case studies that focus on the importance of defining health settings so that health education outcomes can be achieved through selection and application of desired strategies and skills.

To accomplish these goals, we have organized the book into four sections, in which we examine background and theory (Chapters 1–4); settings, skills, and outcomes for health education practice (Chapters 5–8); a case analysis of three health education programs (Chapter 9); and an overview of the evolving roles of health educators—past, present, and future (Chapter 10).

We begin with a chapter reviewing the importance and significance of health education to the health field. The second chapter defines health and education and links these terms into an evolving definition of health education. Chapter 3 assesses the status of health on a worldwide basis and asks, What needs to be changed? It also critiques the current health care system in the United States and offers a model of health care that we feel is part vision and part immediate necessity. In Chapter 4, we define the concept of health education as change through the process of education, and we develop and illustrate a theoretical model for four types of health education change. This chapter also discusses the effects of social values on choices of goals and strategies for change, and it guides the student through the ethical dilemmas inherent in the role of change agent.

Chapters 5, 6, 7, and 8 offer a theoretical model for specific health education practice, based on an analysis of settings, skills, and outcomes. Chapter 5 explores the nature of health education practice, provides an operational definition of health education, and describes the dimensions and determinants of health education programs. Chapter 6 defines the settings for health education. Chapter 7 links settings to specific skills necessary for practice by examining the application of these skills in both formal and informal education and in program planning and evaluation within appropriate settings. Chapter 8 is divided into two sections: the first relates these settings to specific outcomes, which then become a means of defining health problems amenable to health education interventions; and the second provides a discussion of evaluation as a means of measuring the success or failure of health programs.

Chapter 9 illustrates how to translate theory into practice. Three case studies of health education programs are examined for this purpose. The analysis of each case study is based on criteria that will help students learn to use the educational change model as a diagnostic tool in determining the most appropriate educational change strategy to pursue with a particular problem. The analyses illustrate the manner in which each setting defines both the problem and the possible health education interventions. For each case study of a determined health problem, it will be apparent that the type of setting will define the specific outcome, which in turn will determine the health education skills that are required. Final elements of practice include assessing each case study in terms of the planning and implementation of the program; the conduct, organization, and evaluation of the program; and the degree of community involvement.

The final chapter of the book presents an overview of the profession of health education. In Chapter 10, the roles, activities, and functions of the health educator are examined in terms of their historical development, their effect on contemporary practice, and their future directions. Future trends are delineated for six major areas of practice, including primary care and health maintenance organizations, hospital and clinical settings, and occupational and community health settings. We then examine the issues of professional education, role delineation, and credentialing, which continue to arise from the evolving field of health education practice. We conclude this chapter with some reflections of our own about the outlook for health education in the next decade and a half.

We believe this text will be a valuable learning asset for two groups of students. The first group includes undergraduate and graduate students who are preparing themselves for a career in the field of health care and need to know what health education is, how it is practiced, and how this knowledge can be useful to them in their area of specialization. The second group of students includes those who are preparing themselves for a career as health education specialists. We believe that we have presented both of these groups with a clear, concise guide to the field. Others who will find the book of value are the numerous practitioners who consider health education an important aspect of their work: nurses, physicians, social workers, nutritionists, environmentalists, and other health professionals. For these practitioners, this book will be a comprehensive guide that relates issues of health and health delivery to health education, theory, and practice.

We wish to acknowledge our colleagues, past and present, whose values, attitudes, and ideas have influenced us in writing this text. For their thoughtful reading and comments on a preliminary draft of the manuscript, we are grateful to Joseph E. Balog of the University of South Carolina, Lorraine G. Davis of the University of Oregon, Karen Glanz of Temple University, Michael L. Jackson of Western Illinois University, and Alice E. Miller of Southern Illinois University. In addition, we are indebted to Lansing Hays, the health education editor for Mayfield Publishing Company, who encouraged us to proceed from an idea to a completed manuscript. We also would like to thank Merle Rockwell for her numerous editorial comments and suggestions, which have improved the readability of the text. We wish especially to acknowledge the many students in public health whose comments on this manuscript have proved to be an invaluable aid in clarifying and recording our ideas.

Ira J. Bates
Alvin E. Winder

INTRODUCTION TO HEALTH EDUCATION

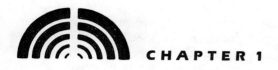

CHAPTER 1

The Challenge: Influencing Health Behaviors and Lifestyles in a Pluralistic Society

In the pantheon of American values, health's only serious rival for supremacy is education. When both values are coupled, as in the matter of health education, we are surely in the presence of a good which is deemed highly desirable in all quarters of American society. We are apparently committed to the idea that an optimally healthy nation requires not only well-trained medical personnel and modern medical facilities but also a citizenry which has positive attitudes toward medical care and knows enough about the symptoms of disease to know when to call upon that care.

If any advances are to be made in reducing illness and increasing longevity, it will apparently be accomplished by motivating masses of individuals to seek medical care before acute illness is already at hand. We are therefore entering a historical period in which the individual and his relationship to the system of medical care becomes of great importance.

Peter H. Rossi, Former Director,
National Opinion Research Center
(Feldman, 1966, p. v)

For a long time, Americans have recognized that our individual personal health behaviors have great effects on the society in which we live. We have witnessed and measured these effects in terms of unnecessary human suffering, numbers of disabilities and premature deaths, increased treatment costs for illnesses, productive time lost because of illness, and deterioration in the overall quality of life. Only recently, however, has enough evidence been available to document the specific results of what some authors now refer to as personal health "mis-behaviors" (Knowles, 1976). Today, enough people appear to be sufficiently concerned about these problems to do something about them.

Yet to change the behaviors of large numbers of individuals is, at best, difficult. John H. Knowles has stated the problem clearly: "Prevention of disease means forsaking the bad habits which many people enjoy—overeating, too much drinking, taking pills, staying up at night, engaging in promiscuous sex, driving too fast, and smoking cigarettes—or, put another way, it means doing things which require special effort—exercising regularly, going to the dentist, practicing contraception, insuring harmonious family life, submitting to screening examinations" (1976, p. 59).

The field of health education has evolved over the past 80 years as the applied social science concerned with the behavioral and lifestyle aspects of human disease. Health education is concerned with the design, conduct, and evaluation of programs that positively influence the health behaviors of individuals, families, small groups, communities, and societies toward adopting healthier lifestyles and improving the quality of life. For example, medical researchers have known for some years that cigarette smoking increases the incidence of lung cancer by approximately 1000 percent and, further, that lung cancer is often fatal. Nevertheless, a 1980 Gallup survey found that 39 percent of the American people claimed not to know that smoking is hazardous to their health. The task of health educators in this instance would be to design and implement programs that would influence behaviors of individuals, small groups, and communities to reduce or stop smoking.

Simply put, the basic approach of health education is that if people can learn about and understand the theories and principles underlying the occurrence of a health problem, they can then learn to alter their own behaviors in ways that will prevent its occurrence. This concept of health education is based on four important assumptions.

1. Theories and principles of disease occurrence can be understood.
2. Appropriate prevention strategies can be developed.
3. Changes in individual and societal health behaviors and lifestyles will affect health status positively.
4. Individuals, families, small groups, and communities can be taught to assume responsibility for their health, which in turn changes their health behaviors and lifestyles.

If students of health education are to be effective, they must have both a working knowledge of these four concepts and an ability to apply them in designing and operating educational programs. Each assumption is based on a number of significant ideas that warrant our review. In the next section, we will discuss each assumption in terms of its development and its relevance to the field of health education.

Theories and Principles of Disease Occurrence

Why does disease occur? The first assumption underlying health education is that a disease process can be understood and explained. Such explanations involve the basic beliefs of a given culture. For centuries, people used only supernatural theories to explain illnesses. Today the method of science provides us with alternative explanations. The story of the evolution of our understanding of disease causation is important because this evolution parallels what Jacob Bronowski has referred to as the "ascent of man": "the development of science as an expression of the special gifts that characterize man and make him preeminent among animals" (1973, p. 20). People's beliefs have always shaped their worlds by defining their thinking. What individuals believe determines what is within their control and what is outside of their control. Their beliefs provide a pivotal point from which they can structure the universe and understand it.

From Panacea to Hygeia: Beliefs About Disease Causation

From the time early men and women first gathered wild berries for food and became ill in the process, individual behavior has been a major determinant of health status. In seeking to understand why they became ill, people developed ideas about causes and effects. If, for example, a man observed that people who ate hemlock berries became ill, he may have decided that it wasn't good to eat hemlock berries. Later, these ideas became rules (don't eat the berries of the hemlock tree), which were passed down to children and to following generations.

Natural Causes. Early people probably understood traumatic causation very well. The effects of accidents or poisonings were obvious, and a person quickly learned how to avoid them. For actions that had an immediate negative effect, people developed rules or customs, based on observations and common sense. (Later we will discuss this concept as the stimulus-response theory of learning.) Such explanations are referred to as *natural causes* of a phenomenon because they could be explained on a rational basis; the relationship between cause and effect was known and understood. "Natural" explanations are important because they increase a person's awareness of the complexity of a phenomenon and identify specific links between individual behavior and the causes of the phenomenon. With this understanding, people could change their behavior in ways that would prevent illness from occurring.

Supernatural Causes.   When a lapse of time occurred between a certain behavior (a cause) and an illness (the effect), people often forgot or could not associate their current condition or illness with their past behavior. If they could not explain their discomfort through natural laws, they turned to supernatural explanations, such as a "spell" or a "hex" placed on them by another person or, more likely, by an evil spirit. Supernatural explanations may lead an individual to accept no responsibility for the course of a disease or illness but, rather, to focus efforts simply on obtaining a "cure." At the same time, this perspective might divert attention from individual behaviors that are, in fact, associated with the problem.

Hygeia and Panacea.   Underlying both natural and supernatural explanations of disease causation are the concepts of prevention and treatment. Basic to the concept of prevention are the assumptions that the individual plays an active, determining role in the process of disease causation and that, by taking certain actions, one can avoid disease occurrence altogether. The concept of treatment or healing comes from the ancient belief that "cures" or "panaceas" can be introduced to limit the disease process and prevent death. Usually a cure was obtained from a member of society who possessed special powers. These designated "priests" were responsible for administering the panacea to those who were ill.

Prototypes for both treatment and prevention can be traced back to Greek culture. According to Greek mythology, Asclepius, the son of Apollo, was a god of healing whose powers were so great that he could bring the dead back to life. When Hades, the god of the dead, jealously complained to Zeus that Asclepius was cheating the kingdom of the dead, Zeus agreed with Hades that Asclepius had violated a basic law of nature by saving mortals from death. Consequently, Asclepius was killed with a thunderbolt. Before he died, however, he gave his healing powers to two of his daughters: Panacea, goddess of healing, who administered medication to the sick, and Hygeia, goddess of health, who taught mortals to live wisely and preserve their bodies.

It was from concepts embodied by these two sisters that we have derived our current understanding of treatment and prevention. *Treatment* refers to the healing process that comes as a "panacea" and is usually obtained from a designated member of society. *Prevention*, which refers to the science of establishing and maintaining health, comes from the term *hygiene*. Both of these concepts are interwoven with the evolution of our beliefs about disease causation. Historically, supernatural explanations of illnesses have prevailed, and remain a very important part of American culture. Only in the past hundred years have we begun to understand disease occurrence enough to move toward more natural explanations. The four theories of disease causation are (1) the evil-spirits theory, (2) the theory of contagion, (3) the germ theory, and (4) the theory of multiple causation.

The Evil-Spirits Theory

The oldest theory of causation, dating from prehistoric times, holds that disease and other mysterious phenomena are the work of invisible, supernatural beings. Early people believed that among the gods who walked the earth and controlled the universe were evil spirits who took over human bodies and caused illnesses. This evil-spirits theory, the belief that every human illness is caused by a devil possessing the body, focuses on symptoms and emphasizes a specific, magical cure. According to this logic, every illness has to be treated; any illness not treated would be fatal.

Throughout history, the search for treatments led people to experiment with extracts derived from many plants and animals, and later with metals. During this empirical era of medical history, practically every known substance was used as a treatment. Cures ranged from physical contact with purported unicorn horns, mandrake roots, and powdered mummies to the potentially more damaging processes of bloodletting and cupping, or of sweating the patient. Emphasis was placed on treatment of symptoms. Bloodletting and exorcism were common procedures in nineteenth-century Europe, for example. In one year alone, 1827, France imported 33 million leeches after its domestic supplies had been depleted. During this time it was also quite common to brutally mistreat the mentally ill in an attempt to force the "evil spirits" out of them.

It was Hippocrates (ca. B.C. 460–377) who first introduced the idea of a rational rather than supernatural explanation of disease occurrence. In his treatise "On Air, Waters and Places," he observed the association of certain types of illnesses with such factors as location, water conditions, climate, eating habits, and housing. Viewing disease as a mass phenomena as well as one affecting individuals, Hippocrates was able also to distinguish between endemic disease (which varied from one locality to another) and epidemic disease (which varied in a point in time). Although he is credited with many ideas that led to modern epidemiologic theory, his teachings had little impact on the popular evil-spirits theory of his time.

The Theory of Contagion

The concept of contagion was the second theory of disease causation to be developed. Oddly enough, it took hundreds of years for people to recognize that some diseases were infectious, or contagious—capable of being transmitted from person to person. Literal interpretation of the Bible, however, taught that "unclean" people should be isolated. By following this religious thought, it was discovered that isolation did reduce incidence of skin diseases such as leprosy. During the thirteenth century, the practice of quarantining arose, based on the idea that isolation might also be effective with other diseases. After the Black Death (bubonic plague), resulted in thousands of deaths in fourteenth-century Europe, the fact that some diseases were infectious could no longer be ignored.

Once the concept of contagion was understood, notions of hygiene arose. When people realized how quickly the Black Death spread, for example, they were reluctant to come into contact with sick people or with anything they touched. Yet ideas of prevention were slow to gain acceptance. Although Ignaz Semmelweis demonstrated in 1847 that the number of women who had died of childbed fever dropped drastically when physicians washed their hands before delivering babies, he failed in his attempt to convince doctors in a Viennese hospital to wash their hands before examinations; it was twenty years before his innovation was accepted.

Based on the theory of contagion, one of the first recorded actions to prevent disease occurred in London in 1854, when a cholera outbreak occurred in the Soho district. A physician named John Snow observed that everyone who became ill drank water from a certain Broad Street pump. When he removed the handle, which prevented people from drinking the water, the cholera epidemic ceased. As a way of explaining what happened, Snow developed the hypothesis that cholera was carried by minute bodies that lived in water contaminated by sewage. These bodies were passed through direct and indirect contact to healthy people, where they multiplied and made these people ill too.

The Germ Theory

The development of the third theory of disease causation, the germ theory, during the 1860's and 1870's marked the first real advance over the evil-spirits theory and the beginning of the conquest of infectious diseases. The germ theory was based on the concept that for every disease there was a single "causal mechanism" that dominated all others. These mechanisms were thought to be minute bodies, previously postulated in the theory of contagion and later defined as microorganisms (e.g., bacteria, fungi, and viruses). According to the germ theory, the development of a disease must be accompanied by the appearance of its mechanism; a major postulate held that this mechanism would be detected in all people with a specific disease, but could not be found in people lacking the disease.

In order to find an effective treatment or prevention using this approach, it was necessary to identify and explain how mechanisms entered and affected the human body. Consequently, proponents of the theory emphasized the search for causal mechanisms through basic research. According to Knowles, the germ theory of disease strengthened the "engineering approach to the human body" and led the medical profession into scientific and technological approaches to disease (1976, p. 68). Demonstrations of the theory by Lister, Pasteur, and Koch between 1860 and

1880 began a public health revolution that ushered in great developments in the science of medicine. As a result of this first public health revolution, human life expectancy would double, from 35 years to 70 years, in less than a century.

The germ theory was "simple, unitary, and compelling: one germ—one disease—one therapy" (Knowles, 1976, p. 68). But, although the theory initiated enormous progress in understanding disease causation, its very simplicity imposed significant limitations on its usefulness for explaining all disease occurrence. The theory ignored factors such as population, personal behavior, and economics. The idea that the "germ" equals the "disease" equals the "treatment" could not account for the complex nature of an occurrence.

It could not account, for example, for the fact that chronic diseases such as hypertension or arthritis were of a different nature than infectious diseases such as measles or polio. Infectious diseases are caused by virulent microorganisms (microorganisms that can produce tissue damage) acquired through exposure to a source of infection (usually another person). Alternatively, chronic diseases result from the activities of microorganisms that remain in our environment for long periods of time. They persist in the body without causing harm under ordinary circumstances; yet they cause disease under conditions of physiological stress.

For example, a physician friend believes that common colds, to a large degree, are psychosomatic. By this he means that we can help to bring upon a cold by allowing ourselves to become ill. Perhaps you have said to yourself, "I can't have a cold now, I'm too busy." The point our friend makes is that the microorganisms that produce respiratory infections already exist in our bodies—but colds result only occasionally. The important difference in explaining chronic disease is that attention must be given to the physiological disturbance (the stress) that converts a latent infection into symptoms of disease. As Rene Dubos has stated, "Throughout nature, infection without disease is the rule rather than the exception (1965, p. 177).

Thus, the basic problem with the germ theory was that it could not explain why some people who were clearly infected did not become ill. In 1893, for example, Koch identified cholera and showed that healthy people excreted large amounts of C. bacillus in their stools. Despite the fact that the C. bacillus has long been known as the mechanism of cholera, even today it has not been possible to produce cholera in human volunteers by feeding them the bacillus, no matter what the dose. At most, a transient diarrhea occurs (Kark, 1974, p. 226).

The Theory of Multiple Causation

To explain disease occurrence in both infectious and chronic diseases, epidemiologists developed the modern theory of multiple causation, by

Figure 1.1 *Web of Causation for Myocardial Infarction*

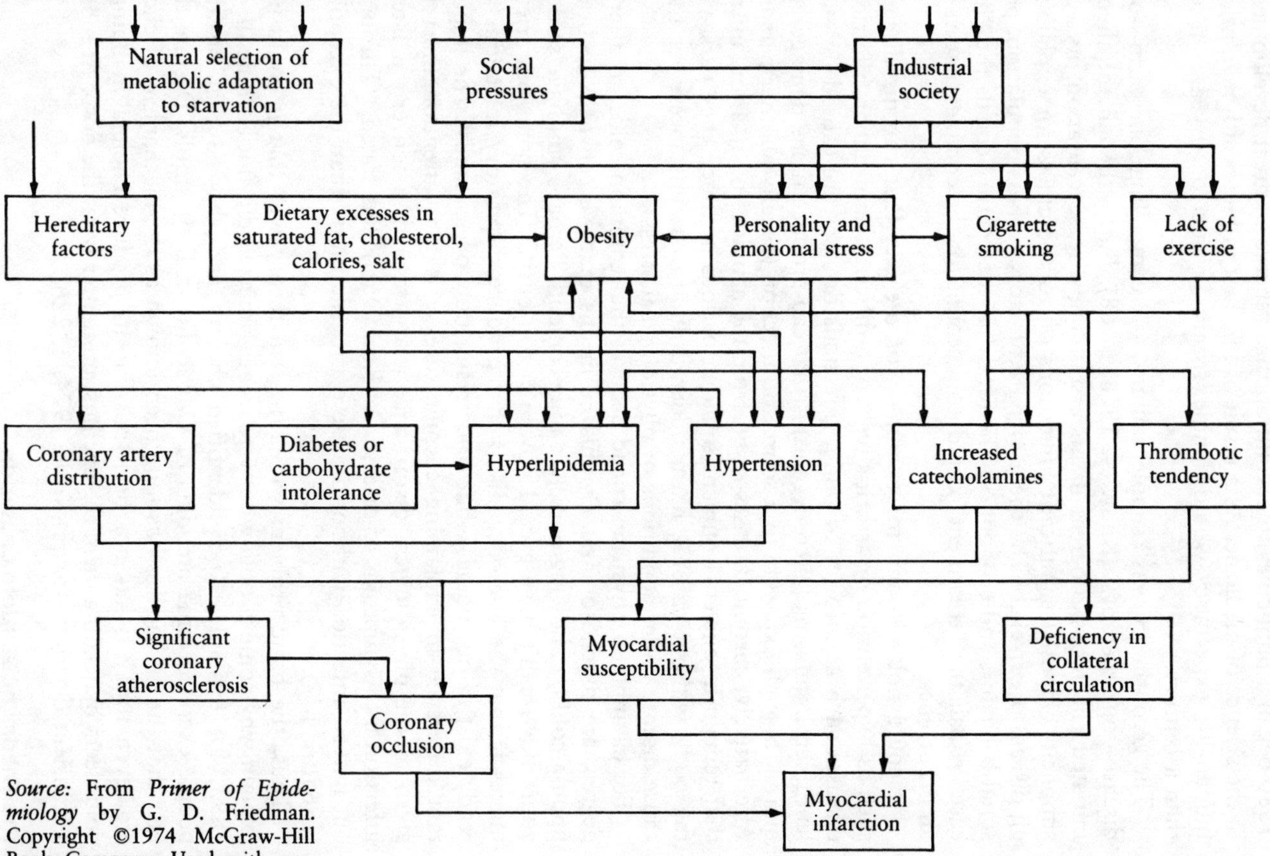

Source: From *Primer of Epidemiology* by G. D. Friedman. Copyright ©1974 McGraw-Hill Book Company. Used with permission of McGraw-Hill Book Company.

observing the process of disease occurrence in several groups of people and comparing differences among these populations over time. The basic idea underlying the theory is that it is impossible to explain a complex occurrence like a disease using a linear, single cause-effect model. Instead, the theory's model of a "web of causation" emphasizes the overall pattern of occurrence and recognizes that numerous factors can be defined as causes. For example, Figure 1.1 shows a web of causation for myocardial infarction, or heart attack. Using this theory it is possible to identify a large number of causes and assess each to determine the most frequent or most important. (This technique is referred to as an epidemiological risk assessment.)

Host-Agent-Environment Relationships. Risk factors can be generally categorized by three types of characteristics: (1) the host (the human being), (2) the agent (the specific cause), and (3) the environment (the conditions where the host and the agent interact). When an imbalance occurs between conditions in the host, the agent, and the environment, a range of host responses may occur (see Figure 1.2, p. 10). For example, an individual exposed to a given cold virus may have (1) no reaction or (2) a physiological reaction (an infection) or (3) a pathologic reaction (exhibiting changes in body tissue) or (4) an illness reaction (showing physical symptoms). According to the theory of multiple causation, in order to understand a specific disease process, it is important to examine host responses to determine (1) the time-intensity gradient and (2) the intensity-frequency relationship for the disease. Donabedian (1973) has provided excellent descriptions of both relationships.

The Time-Intensity Gradient. The concept of a time-intensity gradient is shown in Figure 1.3 (see p. 11), in which time may be defined as hours, days, or years. *Intensity* refers to the degree of host responses, ranging from none to illness or death (or both). The idea is that disease occurs as a process of change that begins with small alterations in the microscopic structure or function of body cells. Over time, the disease begins to have a larger impact until eventually the host feels ill. The disease process may involve a range of courses. It may proceed rapidly, as in a chemical poisoning, or very slowly, until death or recovery. Often, after reaching an acute stage or peak, the disease process wanes, resulting in full recovery or partial disability, as in paralytic polio. Alternatively, a disease such as multiple sclerosis may involve a series of sporadic episodes, each more severe, that may result in progressive disability and death. An important point is that diseases may coexist within a person (usually with adverse effect). Often a person who suffers from a chronic disease does not die from it. What happens is that an acute infection is superimposed upon an individual who is already weakened by a chronic disease. Another point is that

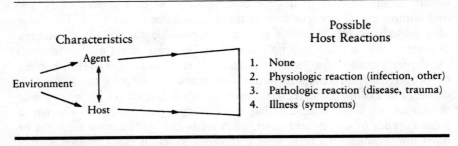

Figure 1.2   *Differences Between Health and Illness*

Source: Adapted from Milton Terris, "Approaches to an Epidemiology of Health," *American Journal of Public Health* 65 (1975): 1038–39.

although the course of any given disease can vary greatly between persons, each disease follows a somewhat predictable course that may be designated its "natural history." This natural history is the course a disease may be expected to follow without intervention or therapy. (Later we will use this concept to develop a strategy of deliberate intervention to interrupt the disease process.)

From Figure 1.3 we can make the following observations about the nature of this time-intensity gradient. (1) The disease may run its entire course without its presence becoming evident. (2) The presence of the disease becomes increasingly evident as the stages progress. (3) Although the stages are not neatly delimited nor orderly in progression, an overall pattern is present.

The Intensity-Frequency Relationships.   Figure 1.4 (see p. 12) shows the second property of a disease: its intensity-frequency relationship. This relationship gives a different perspective of the impact of the disease. Whereas the time-intensity relationship provides a picture of the single host and disease, the intensity-frequency relationship gives a cross-sectional picture of the impact of the disease on the population. In Figure 1.4 the intensity gradient remains the same as it was in Figure 1.3; the horizontal axis shows frequency—the number of people affected.

Interestingly, just as every disease has its own natural history, each disease also has a characteristic frequency distribution by degree of severity (or intensity). This characteristic frequency distribution has been called the "biological gradient of the disease" (Gordon, 1958, p. 337). Significantly, much disease may be submerged below the line at which people feel ill. This has been referred to as "iceberg phenomenon." (Only one-eighth of an iceberg is visible; the rest remains under water.)

Understanding the intensity-frequency relationship helps us to distinguish between infection and disease. Infection may occur without disease

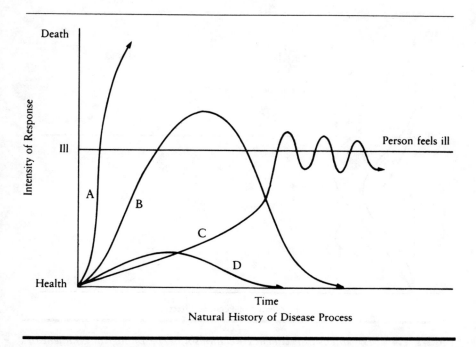

Natural History of Disease Process

Figure 1.3   *The Time-Intensity Gradient of Four Different Disease Processes*

Source: From Avedis Donabedian, *Aspects of Medical Care Administration* (Cambridge, Mass.: Harvard University Press, 1973), by permission of the publisher.

(usually the case), and disease may occur without illness. For example, a large proportion of the adult population have the disease of atherosclerosis, but only a small percentage give evidence of illness. Presumably healthy individuals are often discovered to have tuberculosis or histoplasmosis only because a routine X-ray is taken. Cytological examinations reveal carcinoma of the cervix in numerous healthy women. The concept also explains why transmission of infectious diseases occurs very rapidly. What happens is that people who are infected, but not ill, spread the disease to others, who in turn infect others. Only a few people—the tip of the iceberg—actually become ill, however.

The Development of Prevention Strategies

The second assumption underlying health education is that appropriate prevention strategies can be developed. The idea of prevention is quite simple: it means taking advance measures against something possible or probable. Thus, a prevention strategy is a specific plan for blocking the

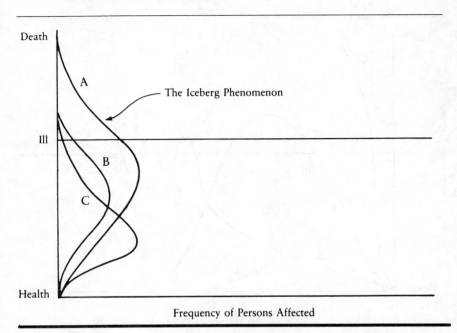

Figure 1.4   *The Intensity-Frequency Relationship: The Biological Gradient of Three Diseases*

Source: From Avedis Donabedian, *Aspects of Medical Care Administration* (Cambridge, Mass.: Harvard University Press, 1973), by permission of the publisher.

occurrence of some event. In those instances in which little, if anything, is known about the event or condition, it is obvious that few actions can be taken to prevent the event from happening. Explaining and understanding why something happens is crucial to our ability to prevent its occurrence.

The Concept of Disease Prevention

Using the concept of the time-intensity gradient—the natural history of disease—Leavell and Clark (1965) developed the model of prevention shown in Figure 1.5. In the model they refer to "prevention" as efforts by health workers to interrupt the natural history of any disease process. The intensity-gradient is represented on the vertical axis by three terms: (1) subclinical or inapparent disease, (2) diagnosis (which usually occurs after a person feels ill), and (3) death (sometimes referred to as the ultimate state of unhealthiness). Following the idea that disease occurs over time, Leavell and Clark identify five phases of a disease: (1) prepathogenesis (before the disease occurs), (2) early pathogenesis (small changes in cells and body tissue), (3) demonstrable but early disease (disease that can be recognized by screening or other diagnostic processes), (4) advanced or

Figure 1.5 *The Natural History of a Disease Process*

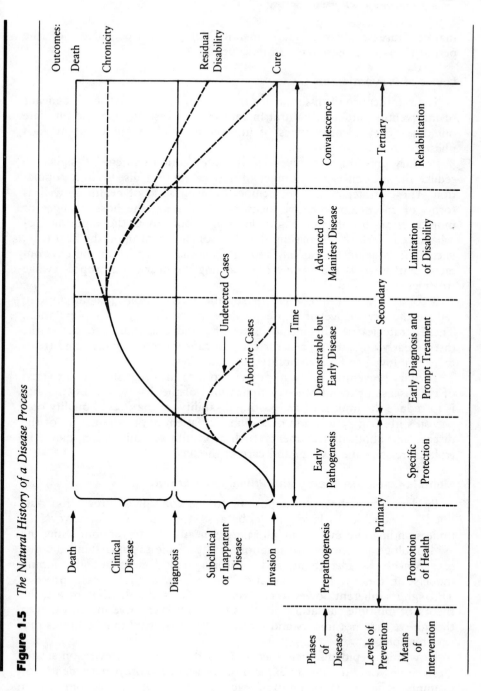

manifest disease (disease clearly identifiable), and (5) convalescence (the period after the disease has run its course).

Levels of Prevention

The significance of this model is that the authors suggest specific means of intervention into the natural history of a disease to alter the ultimate outcome. They identify types of intervention that might occur at each phase of the disease process.

Primary prevention involves specific intervention strategies designed to reduce the incidence (the number of new cases) of a disease in a population. These strategies, which include the promotion of health as well as forms of specific protection, focus on (1) making the host stronger or more resistant to infection (e.g., educating people about the importance of a balanced diet), (2) decreasing the effect of the agent upon the host (e.g., vaccinations against measles), and (3) creating a barrier in the environment that prevents the agent from reaching the host (e.g., proper sewage treatment).

Secondary prevention refers to specific interventions that attempt to reduce the prevalence of a previously existing disease in a population. These strategies usually include screening and casefinding to detect the disease early (e.g., a Pap test for cervical cancer) and diagnosis and treatment employed to limit disability (e.g., diabetes).

Tertiary prevention is the term given to measures that slow the progress of the disease or avoid other complications of the disease process. Its aim is to reduce the impact of an existing disability on the overall quality of a person's life (e.g., education of a diabetic patient about the nature of the disease and about its treatments, such as insulin administration, diet control, exercise, urine testing, and care of the feet).

Multiple-Causation Theory and Primary Prevention

Epidemiologic theory is important to the concept of prevention outlined in Leavell and Clark's model because it provides the framework for understanding and evaluating alternative means of intervention. Using the epidemiological concept of causation, it is possible to understand the disease process by identifying and measuring risk factors and developing models of the "webs of causation" at work in the disease process. Through its inherent power to explain the sources of a disease process, the theory of multiple causation can thus lead to preventative measures, even though we may not understand the exact "mechanism" that produces disease pathology.

How might epidemiologic theory be used to develop prevention strategies? How would the theory explain the cause of motorcycle accidents, for example? The theory of multiple causation is based on recognition that numerous factors can be defined as causes of a disease occurrence. Death resulting from motorcycle accidents may result from speeding, drinking, faulty equipment, poor visibility, heavy traffic, the actions of pedestrians or of other vehicles, driver inexperience, not wearing helmets, or any combination of these factors. Obviously there is no single factor that can be labeled "the cause." It is possible, however, to determine the most frequent or most important causes by using risk-assessment techniques. If one or two of these most frequent causes could be eliminated using specific control measures such as driver training or the use of mandatory safety helmets, then motorcycle fatalities would decrease, but accidents would still happen because of other, albeit lesser, causes. The utility of this theory in primary prevention was clearly demonstrated as early as 1849 by John Snow, when, as you recall, he removed the Broad Street water pump handle and consequently stopped the cholera epidemic (Fox *et al.*, 1970).

The Impact of Changes in Behavior and Lifestyle on Health Status

The third assumption underlying health education is that changes in individual and societal health behaviors and lifestyles will affect health status positively. Although links between peoples' behavior and their health status have long been recognized, the actual measurement of these relationships was begun only in the last 25 years. The problem in establishing these relationships has been twofold. First, it has been (and remains) exceedingly difficult to measure the health status of individuals and populations. Simply put, measures currently available cannot adequately quantify "health status." What they do indicate is "illness status": the degree of disease. Measures that will more adequately quantify "positive health" have yet to be developed. Second, the concepts of health behavior and lifestyle have only recently gained widespread acceptance with the general public and among health professionals, despite the fact that health educators have been talking about these concepts since the 1920's. To fully examine the promise and potential impact of behavior and lifestyle change on health status, the student of health education needs to understand what is meant by these terms and how these concepts have influenced the design of prevention programs.

Health Behaviors and Lifestyles Defined

Behavior is the term used to describe how an individual interacts with other people and his or her environment. *Health behaviors* are ways in which people act, react, and function in particular manners related to their health status. The term *lifestyle* describes "ways of behaving": it refers to the pattern of physical and mental experiences that make up the existence of an individual or that characterize a group. In general, the customs and culture of a group may be referred to as a lifestyle. More specifically, the extent to which a behavior is imbedded in the values, attitudes, and beliefs of an individual determines behavior that is reflected in an individual's lifestyle. This is so because customs are part of the individual's belief system. For example, eating beef is a food preference in American society. Americans believe this food preference reflects both our affluence and our acceptance of a style of British culture. Eating pizza for many Americans is a behavior rather than a custom. It would be much easier for these Americans to give up pizza than it would be to renounce eating beef, because of the beliefs surrounding that food choice. A choice of occupation is a lifestyle decision when the choice is based in part on an individual's beliefs that it is worthwhile to learn the associated skills and that the type of work enhances self-esteem. If the type of job is chosen simply as a way to pay the bills, then the work merely reflects on-the-job behavior.

Table 1.1 lists aspects of human behavior important to disease occurrence (Fox, 1970). The important point about these behaviors is that they are learned ways of thinking, believing, and behaving that are transmitted through the culture of a given population. Although an individual always has a degree of choice in accepting or rejecting these ways of behaving, the behaviors will usually be accepted because they are integral to our culture. By the time we are mature enough to make informed decisions about those lifestyles we personally want to pursue, habits or customs have been so firmly ingrained that it is often very difficult to change them.

Harry Chapin's popular folk song "Cat's in the Cradle" well illustrates this transmission of behaviors. In the song, a father is too busy to have time to talk and play with his young son. The child grows up "wanting to be just like you Dad, just like you." At the end of the song the father wants to spend time with his son, who has since grown up. He finds that the son is too busy, and has become, in fact, just like him. In this instance, the learned behavior had negative overtones. Alternatively, the same situation might have been more positive had the father been more caring in his own behavior.

Beyond the important modeling that occurs within the family structure, society itself exerts powerful forces on its members. External forces such as the ways in which the society distributes its wealth, the amount and type of educational, health, and social services provided, and the availability and range of employment all limit opportunities for the lifestyle choices of individuals. Consider, for example, the occupational choices of two children growing up during the 1950's in different parts of the United States. The son of a coal miner growing up in Appalachia might have had three distinct choices: coal mine, moonshine, or moving down the line (usually to a semiskilled labor job in Ohio, Michigan, or Illinois). In con-

Table 1.1 *Aspects of Human Behavior Related to Disease Occurrence*

Types of Behaviors	Aspects of Disease
Use of water	Intake, quality, quantity, and sources of water
Diet and food handling	Eating habits Food preparation Types of foods consumed Kitchen sanitation Use of milk Use of food additives
Disposal of human wastes	Location and type of toilet Hand washing Use as a fertilizer
Personal hygiene	Bathing Laundering clothing Control of secretions Oral hygiene Protective clothing
Forms of personal contact	Kissing Touching Sexual intercourse
Household hygiene	Sleeping areas General sanitation Food storage
Occupation	Worksite exposure to hazards
Recreation	Use of automobile Travel Outdoor activities
Other behaviors	Smoking Use of drugs Use of physicians

trast, the son of a banker growing up in New York City might have opportunities ranging from joining the family business to going to school to become a physician, artist, or college professor.

Determinants of Health Status

Up to this point we have asked the question "Why does disease occur?" and have used the theory of multiple causation to provide some possible explanations. The question "What determines the health status of a person or a population?" is a somewhat different matter because it involves identifying the factors that come together to result in the person or population becoming healthy or ill at a particular point in time. The health of an individual may vary, for example, depending on the time of day or time of year. At one point the individual may feel well and a moment later feel quite ill. To examine this question for an entire population, we must use an intensity-frequency relationship (see Figure 1.4) because of its cross-sectional view of the population. At any point in time a range of both illnesses and health may be found. Someone may be very ill or near death, while another person may be healthy. When we look at the aggregate at a given point in time, however, there is a frequency distribution of degrees of illness and health that can be quantified in some manner. Some commonly used measures of health status include comparing (1) numbers of living persons versus those who died (e.g., mortality rates), (2) degrees of disability, (3) different types of diseases (e.g., morbidity rates), and (4) degrees of illness (e.g., number of episodes of illness).

The important difference between the two questions we have raised is that if the individual or population has a negative health status (is either ill, or diseased), then they may take actions to improve their status by interrupting the natural history of the condition. For example, many people go to a physician or some other medical provider when they are sick. Others may take over-the-counter drugs or use folk remedies to improve their situation.

To answer the question of what determines the health status of both individuals and populations, Blum (1976) identified four determinants: (1) biological factors, (2) exposure to environmental hazards, (3) access to health services, and (4) lifestyles. How these factors come together to determine health status is shown in the formula

$$HS = (f)\ E + AcHs + B + Ls$$

where HS equals health status, a dependent variable; (f) equals some combination or function of a series of independent variables; E equals hazards in the environment; $AcHs$ equals access to health services; B equals human biological factors; and Ls equals behavioral or lifestyle change.

Like the theory of multiple causation, this model does not focus on single cause-effect, linear relationships. Instead, health status is seen as an outcome (a dependent variable) with four major determinants (independent variables). For example, a high rate of lung cancer (a measure of health status, HS) in a community could be explained using this model as the interaction of exposures to certain environmental hazards, such as asbestos or cigarette smoke (E); access to health services, such as the ability to pay for services or the availability of medical providers to diagnose and treat the problem ($AcHs$); biological factors, such as a family history of cancer or the presence of other diseases (B); and lifestyle factors, such as a history of smoking behavior, type of occupation, and length of time worked (Ls).

The assumption underlying the model is that if we can change the nature of any of these independent variables, improvements in health status will result. At the level of primary prevention, such changes might include air pollution programs to reduce exposure of the population to certain chemicals, programs to help people stop smoking, or provision of financial assistance to people employed in high-risk occupations so that they might change their employment. At the secondary-prevention level, interventions might include screening programs to identify individuals at risk, special laboratory procedures to help in diagnosis, or advanced treatment procedures or educational programs designed to help people with lung cancer to understand the treatment process. Tertiary-level prevention programs might include assistance to the family of an individual with lung cancer or educational programs for patients to help them deal with the possibility of their own death.

A significant point is that our understanding of these determinants of health status has evolved over the past hundred years, just as our beliefs about disease causation have changed. These changing ideas have helped to shape both the nature of intervention programs and the public's response to such programs. For example, the first public health revolution, which we will discuss in the next section, emphasized environmental concerns (E) as the answer to improved health status. Later, in the 1950's, emphasis shifted to access to health services $(AcHs)$ as the way to better health. More recently, the second public health revolution has been based on the thesis that lifestyles (Ls) of people should change if health is to improve. The following review of these movements should provide some more historical perspective about the way in which beliefs have influenced the development of health programs.

Hygela Emerges: The First Public Health Revolution

The first public health revolution, which began in the late nineteenth century and continued through the 1950's, was for the most part a struggle against the great epidemic diseases: cholera, plague, smallpox, yellow fever, typhus, tuberculosis, and polio. Basing their attack on these infectious diseases on the notion that environmental factors greatly affected health status, health professionals used the primary prevention strategies of (1) major sanitation measures (chlorination of water, treatment of raw sewerage, and regulation of water and sewerage); (2) development of effective vaccines used in mass immunizations (polio, smallpox); (3) regulation of the food supply (pasteurization of milk, inspection of food-handling establishments); (4) improvements in nutrition (availability of beef and grain products in cities); and (5) provision of adequate housing (homes heated by coal, oil, and gas).

By the early 1950's those public health control strategies initiated at the turn of the century began to have a profound effect on the health of the

American population, in terms of both numbers of lives saved and the
general quality of life. Between 1900 and 1977 deaths resulting from major acute diseases (including influenza, pneumonia, diphtheria, tuberculosis, and gastrointestinal infections) declined from 580 to 30 for every
100,000 Americans. Today the infectious diseases of the 1900's account
for only 1 percent of those who die before age 75. The overall death rate
has been reduced from 17 per 1,000 people per year to less than 9 per
1,000. These changes, in turn, have resulted in a much older population.
In qualitative terms, too, there has been a shift in interest from prevention
of death to an emphasis on health and the quality of life.

A Return to Panacea: The Medicated Society

Although the advances of the first public health revolution were interpreted as great victories for the public health movement, they were, more
importantly, seen as victories for science and technology. Accomplish-
ments such as the development of polio and measles vaccines, the emergence of antibiotics and other "miracle drugs," and the development of
effective surgical treatments led to an "engineering approach" to the human body. This approach, which emphasized biological factors (B), was
initially so effective that some people believed a medical utopia was only a
few years away. The answer, it seemed, was investment of money into
biomedical research—basic research into the functions of the human body.
The rationale was that once the human body was better understood, the
causes of diseases would be known and preventive strategies could be developed that would then be disseminated throughout the medical care system. Thus, given sufficient technology, all of the American people could
receive treatments for their illnesses.

This belief that science and technology could solve health and social
problems was so great that it led the World Health Organization (WHO)
in 1950 to optimistically define health as "a state of complete physical,
mental and social well-being and not merely the absence of disease or in-
firmity." In 1965 Rene Dubos countered this view in his book *Mirage of
Health*. Public health workers, Dubos wrote "face a peculiar intellectual
dilemma. On the one hand they are professionally committed to the doc-
trine that it is possible to create a world free of disease; they must function as if they believe in a Medical Utopia. On the other hand, experience
teaches them that as soon as one disease is rooted out, another springs up
to take its place. . . . Public health workers know that the 'positive health'
evoked by the WHO definition is at best a mirage that can never be
reached, and perhaps nothing more than a will-o-the-wisp that may lead
its followers into the swamps of unreality" (p. 23).

The "experience" to which Dubos referred had taught that, although
death rates for the infectious diseases had been drastically reduced, these
diseases were being replaced by the modern epidemics of coronary heart

disease, cancer, hypertension, diabetes, arthritis, alcoholism, accidents, suicides, and homicides. In 1979, for example, the United States Surgeon General reported that "cardiovascular disease, including both heart disease and stroke, accounts for roughly half of all deaths. Cancer accounts for another 20 percent. Accidents exact a fearsome toll of death and disability among young people." The Surgeon General's Report also noted that the proportion of mortality from major chronic diseases such as heart disease, cancer, and stroke, had increased more than 250 percent since the 1900's (p. vii).

Despite such cautions, the followers of Panacea reemerged during the 1950's and gained strength through the mid-1970's, bolstered by their belief in the power of science and technology. This 30-year period saw unprecedented growth in the medical care system: the number of physician specialties expanded, hospital and tertiary-care treatment facilities increased, and new modalities of treatment such as hyperbaric chambers, radium and cobalt therapy, and CAT-scanners were developed. The growth of services was so phenomenal that it led Somers (1969) to compare the role of the hospital in modern America to that of the cathedral in medieval Europe. Both were complex social institutions "serving simultaneously a variety of purposes—welfare center, object of civic pride, major source of employment, market for artists, artisans, and architects, inspirer of saintly deeds and beneficiary of repentant sinners, occasional 'cover-up' for hypocrites and exploiters, source of power, and object of political conflict. Both institutions reflected the values of their day. Both have contained deep internal contradictions" (p. ix).

The commonly accepted assumption underlying the rapid growth of the medical care system was that access to health services (*AcHs*) primarily determined health status. It was believed that there existed a strictly limited quantity of morbidity, and that more widespread treatment would result in a reduction of subsequent sickness rates. Consequently, as effective therapy reduced morbidity, costs would logically decline. Given this rationale, the central issue became one of universal access to treatment: How could comprehensive personal health services be organized, financed, and delivered in such a way as to ensure that everyone had an opportunity to receive them?

Answers to this question came in the mid 1960's with the passage by Congress of Medicare, Medicaid, Regional Medical Programs (RMP), and Comprehensive Health Planning (CHP) legislation. These programs were designed to finance the health care system in order to provide care for those who could not afford it (those over age 65 and the medically indigent) and to reorganize the system in order to improve the distribution of services. In the push to remove financial barriers to access, however, most advocates denied or failed to recognize the critical relationship between financing and organization. It was not until the late 1960's, when costs were spiraling, that this key link was fully appreciated. As Somers (1976) explained, although "the billions of new money produced by Medicare and Medicaid and government guaranteed full reimbursement to providers" and "forced a desirable upgrading of quality among inferior hospitals, nursing homes, and home health services," almost all of these institutions "were affected by the heady atmosphere of easy money. Most doctors strove to become specialists, and ordinary hospitals strove to become tertiary care centers. All wanted to be self-sufficient." As a result, "primary care and family practice seemed on the verge of disappearing. . . . By the end of the 1960's, patients were complaining that their care was more fragmented and more complicated to obtain than ever before. It was also clear that the fragmentation was contributing to the cost spiral" (p. 57).

Disappointment with Panacea

According to Knowles (1976), "acute, curative technology-dependent medicine reached its apogee in the 1960's and, as expectations rose, so did the cost" (p. 59). From 1950 to 1975 total health expenditures rose from $12 billion to $118.5 billion, a 988 percent increase with an annual average of 9.6 percent. In the same 25-year period the proportion of the Gross National Product spent on health increased 80 percent, reaching 8.3 percent in 1975. By that year the federal government was spending $547 per person for health services, a figure that had been climbing over 10.2 percent a year since 1950.

By the early 1970's Americans were becoming more aware of the distinction between "health" and "medical care." This important difference was lost in the 1960's, when the pursuit of health was identified with professional research, physician care, and more dollars to pay for specialized hospital care. "Care" had come to mean inpatient treatment for the acutely ill. The role of individuals in their own health maintenance was limited to maintaining adequate health insurance coverage, gaining access to a hospital, and visiting a physician for an annual checkup.

In the mid 1970's the consensus based on the premise that medical care was the primary determinant of health status had begun to dissolve. There was a growing conviction that Western societies' reliance on medical care services had become excessive, and that the diversion of resources to exotic high-technology procedures was socially wasteful. Moreover, despite the vast increase in health care expenditures and improved access to care, the health of the American people as measured by illness, disability, and premature deaths showed little, if any, improvement. After a half century of steady and dramatic improvement, in the 1960's the total death rate for the United States had ceased to decline. Between 1960 and 1973 it remained almost stable, ranging from 9.7 to 9.3 per 1,000 persons.

For many people it appeared as if therapeutic medicine had almost reached a point of diminishing return. The 12 to 15 percent increase per year in the $100 billion health care bill (even after being discounted for inflation) was apparently having a marginal effect on health status. In 1974 the economist Victor Fuchs, in his book *Who Shall Live?*, provided the scholarly documentation for this point of view. "Health levels," Fuchs wrote, "are usually not related in any important degree to differences in medical care. Over time, the introduction of new medical technology has had a significant impact on health, but when we examine differences among populations, other socioeconomic and cultural variables are much more important than differences in the quantity or quality of medical care" (p. 16). To emphasize his point, Fuchs contrasted the health status of people living in Nevada and Utah, "states that enjoy about the same levels of income and medical care and are alike in many other respects." In spite of these similarities, however, the levels of health in these two states differ enormously: "The inhabitants of Utah are among the healthiest individuals in the United States, while the residents of Nevada are at the opposite end of the spectrum. . . . What, then, explains the huge differences?" The answer, Fuchs concluded, "almost surely lies in the different lifestyles of the residents of the two states" (p. 52). Fuchs ended his analysis with a statement that has frequently been quoted to support the need for changes in lifestyles. Noting both the critical importance of individual decisions about diet, exercise, and smoking and the relevance of collective decisions about environmental matters such as pollution, he declared that "the greatest current potential for improving the health of the American people is to be found in what they do or don't do to and for themselves" (p. 55).

Relationships Between Lifestyles and Health Status

Although the role of lifestyle was thus believed to be associated with health status, evidence of this relationship was limited in the early 1970's. The first solid evidence that the lifestyles of individuals have a substantive impact on their health status was published in 1972 by Lester Breslow, dean of the School of Public Health, University of California, and N. B. Belloc of the Human Population Laboratory, California Department of Public Health (1972, pp. 413–421). In this landmark study, nearly 7,000 adults were followed for five and a half years. The research showed that life expectancy and better health were significantly related to seven simple, yet basic, health habits:

1. Three meals a day at regular times and no snacking
2. Breakfast every day
3. Moderate exercise two or three times a week
4. Adequate sleep (seven or eight hours a night)
5. No smoking

6. Maintenance of moderate weight

7. No alcohol or use of alcohol only in moderation

Breslow and Belloc found, for instance, that a 45-year-old man who practiced up to three of these habits had a life expectancy of 21.6 years (to age 67), whereas a man who practiced six or seven of them had a life expectancy of 33.1 years (to age 78). The authors explained that "the magnitude of this difference of more than 11 years is better understood if we consider that the increase in the life expectancy of white men in the United States between 1900 and 1960 was only 3 years." Their conclusion: "that certain common habits of daily life, called good health habits, are positively related to physical health status" and, further, that the relationship of these habits is cumulative—"those who reported all or many of the good practices were in better physical health, even though older, than those who followed fewer such habits. These relationships were independent of economic status" (pp. 67–81). Indeed, the physical health status of those who practiced all seven habits was similar to persons who were 30 years younger but who followed none of these practices.

To illustrate the impact of lifestyle on the health of the American population, the 1979 Surgeon General's Report estimated that "as much as half of U.S. mortality in 1976 was due to unhealthy behavior or lifestyle; 20 percent to environmental factors; 20 percent to human biological factors; and only 10 percent to inadequacies in health care" (p. 9). In another study, Gori and Richter (1978) described lifestyle changes that could be accomplished by the American people and estimated the probable impact of these changes on major causes of death (see Table 1.2). Their data, Gori and Richter summarized, clearly indicated "that an even more determined and massive action is required in respect to diet, smoking, alcohol and drug abuse, and automobile and occupational safety." The authors noted too, however, that the course of action they outlined "presents greater difficulties than do simple engineering approaches to environmental preservation, because it calls for a conscious commitment to modify lifestyles and to reconsider social and economic conventions such as the preoccupation with continuing economic growth and the concept of dutiful labor" (p. 1124).

Hygeia Reemerges: Beginning the Second
Public Health Revolution

Interestingly, it was leadership from another country that pushed emphasis on lifestyles into the forefront of public health policy. In 1974, under the direction of Marc Lalonde, Minister of National Health and Welfare, the government of Canada published *A New Perspective on the Health of Canadians*. It introduced into public policy the concept (previously described by Blum, 1976) that all causes of death and disease had

Table 1.2 *Influence of Enviromental and Lifestyle Factors on Mortality*

Factor	Major Cardio-vascular and Renal Diseases	Malignant Neoplasms	Accidents, Motor Vehicle and Other	Respira-tory Diseases	Diabetes Mellitus
		Cause of Death			
Smoking	VH	VH	L	VH	VL
Diet	VH	VH	VL	VL	VH
Occupational hazards	VL	L	VH	H	VL
Alcohol abuse	L	L	VH	L	L
Drug abuse	VL	VL	H	VL	VL
Radation hazards	VL	L	VL	VL	VL
Air and water pollution	VL	VL	VL	L	VL
		Number of Premature Deaths			
In 1973	395,000	90,000	44,000	16,000	24,000
In 2000*	595,000	127,000	71,000	33,000	30,000

VH = very high impact (more than 30%)
 H = high impact (20–30%)
 M = medium impact (10–20%)
 L = low impact (5–10%)
VL = very low impact (less than 5%)

Note: *If current trends remain unchanged.

Source: Adapted from G. B. Gori and B. J. Richter, "Macroeconomics of Disease Prevention in the United States," *Science* 200 (1978): 1124 – 30.

four contributing elements: (1) inadequacies in the existing health care system, (2) behavioral factors or unhealthy lifestyles, (3) environmental hazards, and (4) human biological factors.

The central message was that improvements in the environment and in the lifestyles of individuals would be the single most effective means of reducing mortality and morbidity. As a result of this report, the Canadian government began "Operation Lifestyle," which shifted emphasis of its public policies from the treatment to the prevention of illness or, in more positive terms, toward the "promotion of health."

By the mid 1970's the new advocates of Hygeia had gathered enough forces to gain some attention within the United States government. In

1972, for example, the President appointed a Task Force on the Education of the Public. Two years later the National Health Planning and Resource Development Act of 1974 specified public health education as one of the nation's priorities, and in 1976 the passage of P.L. 94-317 established the Office of Health Information and Health Promotion under the Assistant Secretary of Health in the Department of Health Education and Welfare.

However, it was the publication in 1979 of the first Surgeon General's Report on Health Promotion and Disease Prevention that proclaimed the second public health revolution. Entitled *Healthy People,* this watershed document's purpose was clear: "to encourage a second public health revolution in the history of the United States." The thesis of the report was that "further improvements in the health of the American people can and will be achieved—not alone through increased medical care and greater expenditures—but through a renewed national commitment to efforts designed to prevent disease and promote health" (p. 7). Proclaiming that "prevention is an idea whose time has come," the report went on to say that "we have the scientific knowledge to begin to formulate recommendations for improved health. And, although degenerative diseases differ from their infectious disease predecessors in having more—and more complex—causes, it is now clear that many are preventable" (p. 10).

The keys to prevention, according to the Surgeon General's Report, were not only the "actions decision makers in the public and private sectors can take to promote a safer and healthier environment" but also the "actions individuals can take for themselves" (p. 9), including

1. Elimination of cigarette smoking
2. Reduction of alcohol abuse
3. Moderate dietary changes to reduce intake of excess calories, fat, salt, and sugar
4. Moderate exercise
5. Periodic screening (at intervals determined by age and sex) for major disorders such as high blood pressure and certain cancers
6. Adherence to speed laws and the use of seat belts

Changing Health Behaviors and Lifestyles

The recommendation of individual action for better health by the Surgeon General's Report touched on what is perhaps the most critical assumption underlying the promise of behavioral and lifestyle change: that individuals, families, small groups, and communities can be taught to assume responsibility for their health and that this assumption of responsibility, in turn, brings about changes in their health behaviors and lifestyles. This is the fundamental principle of health education, and it raises a number of important philosophical and practical questions: Does anyone have the right to tell another person what their behavior or lifestyle ought to be, regardless of whether the change would improve the person's health status? Is it possible to achieve desirable social ends without sacrificing individual freedoms? How can individual or group behavior be changed while reinforcing individual responsibility? If health education is to be understood as a profession and a discipline, each of these questions needs to be placed in perspective.

The Challenge of Health Education

The field of health education emerged from the larger science of public health, which has as its purpose "the diagnosis and treatment of the body politic" (MacGavern, 1955). Consequently, health education shares the philosophical perspective of public health, the main tenet of which is that planned social change is both useful and desirable when it promotes the public good. All public health workers, to some degree, believe that regulation of individual behavior and social control of the population is necessary to protect the health of the commonwealth. Because all planned social change implies a commitment to change current ways of doing things, this philosophy means that people are asked (in a democratic society) or told (in a totalitarian society) to alter their behaviors or their lifestyles for the larger "public good."

The field of health education has evolved over the past 80 years as the applied social science concerned with behavioral and lifestyle aspects of human disease. Since its inception, health educators have recognized the important link between lifestyle and health status. Health education as an applied discipline utilizes principles from the fields of education, social psychology, anthropology, sociology, demography, communications, economics, political science, and other related disciplines to create change. These changes may occur at a variety of levels: changes that result in individuals shifting from one behavior to another, changes in which individuals alter their lifestyles, changes that restructure and refocus social institutions, and changes that bring about the fundamental transformation of a society's prevailing economic or sociocultural values.

The basic challenge of health education is to find appropriate ways to influence individual behaviors and lifestyles in a pluralistic, democratic society. From a philosophical perspective, the question facing both public health and health education is, How do we maintain the individual's freedom and at the same time achieve desirable social ends? Conversely, How do we change individual or group behaviors and at the same time reinforce individual responsibility? Answers to these questions, in a democratic society, involve people using knowledge and expressing attitudes and values that they have learned in order to make decisions that affect their own lives. It is the premise that individuals can be taught to become competent decision makers that forms the basis for the practice of health education.

The field of health education is concerned with creating voluntary change that affects health status. As a profession, it has rejected the prescriptive "should do or ought to do" approaches of traditional public health and has, instead, developed alternative approaches that emphasize humanistic behavioral and lifestyle changes through educational processes. These approaches "enhance the individual's awareness of the options for personal choice and increase his or her competency to translate these choices into action (National Center for Health Education, 1978, p. 14). Although its methods have changed, the purpose of health education has remained steadfast: "The aim of health education is to help people to achieve health by their own actions and efforts. Health education begins therefore with the interests of people in improving their conditions of living, and aims at developing sense of responsibility for their own health betterment as individuals, and as members of families, communities, or governments" (Derryberry, 1952, p. 1).

Critical Issues in Health Education

Given that the basic challenge of health education is to find appropriate ways to influence individual behaviors and lifestyles in a pluralistic, democratic society, it is obvious that this challenge raises numerous questions that must be addressed by health educators. These questions will provide our agenda for the rest of this book. In Chapter 2, for example, we will look at these basic questions: What is health? How do we learn, and What constitutes education? What is the link between health and education, and how do we define health education as a process? In Chapter 3 we will examine some ideological comments about health and ask, What needs to be changed? To formulate an answer, in Chapter 4 we will establish perspectives on the meaning of change and the function of health educators in the change process. Then, in Chapters 5 through 8 we will define health education practice by looking at the following questions: What is an operational definition of health education? What are settings for health education practice? What are the essential competencies of health educators? And, What outcomes are expected from health education programs? Finally, in Chapters 9 and 10 we will place the field of health education into the real world by asking, How is a health education program organized and carried out? Further, what are the specific roles, activities, and functions of health educators?

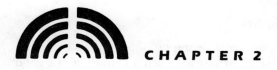

CHAPTER 2

Health, Education, and Health Education: How Are They Related?

We are embarking on a journey that has as its goal an understanding of health education as both a body of knowledge and a field of practice. Our concern, however, is with the journey itself, for we believe that understanding is a process that comes not only with acquired knowledge but also with the provision of opportunities for the learner to critically evaluate the ideas and beliefs to be encountered on the natural course of the trip.

In this chapter we have mapped some of the difficult terrain that you must pass through in the initial stages of your journey. There is great difficulty, for example, in defining health education. Many champions have been called forth to accomplish this task. To some, it has seemed simple enough, and they have accordingly produced suitable definitions, stepping forward to accept the rewards of a grateful public. None has fully succeeded.

Our first task is to obtain an adequate definition of health. Our second task will be to examine educational theory in order to determine how people learn. We will then proceed to clarify the links between health and education and, finally, to outline a theory of health education that is both consistent with what you have learned on your journey and useful in guiding health education practice.

Toward a Definition of Health

We now take our first steps toward a definition of health. To begin, we
might say that health is the absence of disease. Such a definition is a good
start because, to the thoughtful individual, it raises a number of questions.
What is disease? Why do people get sick? Can we prevent disease? Why
don't people get sick more often? Three contemporary approaches to a
definition of health attempt to answer these and other questions. We will
call them (1) the health-disease dichotomy, (2) the continuum model of
health and illness, and (3) the systems view of health.

The Health-Disease Dichotomy

The health-disease dichotomy is an elaboration on the idea that health
is the absence of disease. Those health professionals who believe in the
health-disease dichotomy define health primarily in terms of a clinical
model or a public health model of health and illness.

The Clinical Model.   We have encountered the clinical model when we enter a physician's office and wait for the doctor to determine whether we
are sick or well. Table 2.1 presents us with a Aaron Antonovsky's repre-
sentation of this model as it is viewed by lay persons and health care providers (1979). The model works as follows: You enter the health system,
and a provider, usually a physician, asks "What hurts?" Your complaint
is noted as a symptom. Tests are performed to relate your symptom to
some kind of organic sign. "Your throat hurts; may I look? Ah yes—red
with white spots." You are then diagnosed as being diseased and assigned
to one of the conventional categories whose ultimate listing can be found
in the International Classification of Diseases. Presumably, treatment will
then be prescribed.

The clinical model overlooks some important distinctions that most of
us can easily relate to our own experiences. First, on any given day, many
of us may feel bad in general—a condition we frequently tolerate as long
as the period of discomfort is relatively short and we are not incapaci-
tated. Second, we may at a given time announce to ourselves or another
that we are sick. At times a friend will say, "You don't look well," or
"You look like you have the flu." These remarks are not usually an invita-
tion to go see the doctor or to enter the health care system. Usually they
are a sign that someone recognizes your discomfort and suggests you take
care of yourself, get rest, apply home remedies, and accept, for the moment, a less stressful and more dependent role. Should you visit a physician, however, you will be labeled a patient. Like so many others who
enter the physician's office, you will have entered the health care system.
And like so many others who have traveled the same path, you will find
that because your complaints fail to fit the diagnostic categories of the

Table 2.1   *The Clinical Model*

A. A nonpatient
   1. Healthy
   2. Sick
      a. Feeling bad in general
      b. Sick with a particular diagnosis of a particular "disease" as defined by oneself or another layperson

B. A patient
   1. Diseased
      a. With signs sufficiently clear to allow subclassification as
         (1) A case of disease X
         (2) A case of disease Y and/or
         (3) A case of disease n
      b. With insufficient signs to allow specific disease subclassification
   2. Not diseases: malingerer, crock, hypochondriac or emotionally disturbed person

Source: Aaron Antonovsky, *Health, Stress, and Coping* (San Francisco: Jossey-Bass, 1979).

International Classification of Diseases, you will probably be prescribed a sedative and dismissed with the hope that your current stress will abate or that the sedative action will make further demands on the physician's time unnecessary.

The Public Health Model.   A second approach that defines health, the public health model, differs from the clinical model in that its concern is with group rather than with individual pathology. The aim of the public health model is to control environments and prevent pathology. Just as diagnosis serves the clinical model in the detection of disease, epidemiological analysis serves the public health model in the detection of pathology in groups. Epidemiology serves both as the scientific discipline for determining the incidence and prevalence of diseases in the population and as a means for seeking to understand the causes leading to their presence. An analysis of historic trends in health and disease provides strong supporting data for the public health model. For example, nearly all the major infectious diseases of the Middle Ages had all but disappeared by the time their etiology, prevention, or therapy was understood. Their ebb is usually ascribed to improved living conditions—notably better nutrition, clean food and water, better education, safer employment, and better housing. Winkelstein (1976) makes a clear case that this significant drop in mortality rates had little to do with the development of antibacterial and antidisease treatment.

The Problem with the Health-Disease Dichotomy. A significant problem with both the public health and the clinical models is their division of people into the categories of healthy or sick. As we noted in Chapter 1, recently many health professionals have promoted a shift in emphasis from the treatment of disease to the maintenance of health: the 1979 Surgeon General's Report, *Healthy People,* specified the "promotion of health" as the aim of public policy in its approach to the health care system. The conceptualization of health, however, is even more difficult than the conceptualization of pathology. Is health simply the absence of disease? Cochrane (1972) found that if you collect a great many biological measurements from a group of people, they do not fall into a bimodal distribution of sick and healthy. Instead, they fall on a distribution curve. At what point on the curve does a clinician decide that a systolic blood pressure reading should be categorized as indicating hypertension? Or, given a distribution of blood sugar levels, at what point does the clinician say a person has diabetes?

Susser (1974) has provided a useful guide for pursuing this problem of conceptualization. He divides health into three levels: the somatic, the personal, and the social. This model is best illustrated if we refer to illness. Assume that X has recently broken his leg. His health is impaired. The term *somatic level* refers to the degree of impairment of a part of his body: X has a fracture of a bone in his leg and cannot walk. The *personal level* (or psychological level) refers to the individual's feelings of discomfort: X complains that his leg aches and is very painful when he tries to move it. The *social level* refers to the individual's assumption of a sick or handicapped role in society: X has visited a physician who set his leg and prescribed bed rest; he has called his place of employment, stated that he is sick and is home in bed, where his wife can take care of him. If X had not broken his leg, he would have no bodily impairment. He would say that he feels fine and would go to work and independently take care of himself. He would be healthy. The strength of this conceptualization is that it defines health and disease along the three coordinates: somatic, personal (psychological), and social.

The Continuum Model of Health and Illness

An alternative model to the health-disease dichotomy, and one that satisfies the data supplied by the distribution curve of physiological functioning discussed by Cochrane, is Antonovsky's conceptualization of a health-disease continuum (1979). Although each of Susser's axes—somatic, personal, and social—can be seen as a continuum, with health at one end and malfunction at the other, his emphasis is on pathogenesis. Antonovsky, in contrast, has been concerned with the question of how we remain healthy, especially in light of "the ubiquity of pathogens—microbiological, chemical, physical, psychological, social, and cultural"—in our environment (p. 13). Why, he wondered, weren't people constantly dying, succumbing to this bombardment of pathogens?

Terming the capacity to remain healthy "salutogenesis," Antonovsky proposed the salutogenic model of health, based on a continuum with ease (health) at one end and disease at the other. What are the origins of health? According to this model, they are to be found in what Antonovsky calls a person's sense of coherence. An individual who has a good sense of coherence would be at the ease end of the ease-disease continuum. An individual who has a poor sense of coherence would be at the disease end of the continuum. Changes in the sense of coherence lead to shifts in position on the ease-disease continuum.

What, then, is the sense of coherence? Antonovsky defines it as "a global orientation that expresses the extent to which one has a pervasive enduring, though dynamic, feeling of confidence that one's internal and external environments are predictable and that there is a high probability that things will work out as well as can be reasonably expected" (p. 10). One's sense of coherence is shaped by the interaction of two major sources—childrearing patterns and social-role complexes—that together provide individuals both with a sense of who they are and how they fit into a given society and also with the significant beliefs and values by which they live. If your self-esteem is high and the beliefs and values you choose as a design for living are well integrated into your personality, supported by your social group, and reflected in your social role, you are then in possession of a strong sense of coherence. The stronger the sense of coherence in individuals and groups, Antonovsky argues, the more adequately persons will cope with the stresses immanent in life and the better are their chances to maintain or improve their health.

We can, in arriving at a more adequate conceptualization of health and illness, borrow from both Susser's and Antonovsky's work and view the healthy individual as one whose balance between health and disease places him or her closer to the health end of each of three axes—somatic, personal (psychological), and social. If theory is to be useful as a means of informing and guiding practice, however, it must be backed up by evidence. And, in fact, researchers have compiled data suggesting, first, that the causes of illness reside in the somatic, psychological, and social environments of humankind and, second, that the imbalance we call disease is a result of the interaction of forces within the somatic, psychological, and social environments of an individual.

Researchers in social epidemiology, for example, have contributed to an understanding of the interactions of all three environments and their effects on illness. Major studies, which include the work of Syme and

Berkman (1976), Jacobs and Ostfeld (1977), Cassel (1974), and Nuckolls, Cassel, and Kaplan (1972), have in common the finding that people placed in highly stressful situations are at risk to become ill. Berkman (1977) proposes that individuals placed in such situations are subject "to powerful socially structured constraints on an individual's ability to maintain enduring and effective social ties" (p. 19).

Working in other disciplines, Wolf and Goodell (1968) and Hinkle and Wolff (1967) have strongly documented the relationship between cultural change and morbidity among American Indian tribes, Bantu natives, and Chinese expatriates living in New York. Wolf and Goodell note that American Indian tribes who were "taken from their homeland and put into reservations within a few miles' distance, in essentially the same physical environment, but in setting of social disorganization," evidenced "a resultant appalling increase in mortality from tuberculosis" (p. 80). A similar result was reported among Bantu natives who were moved from the countryside outside of Johannesburg into the environs of the city (p. 35). As a third example of morbidity and mortality associated with a radical change in physical and social environment, Wolf and Goodell cite the study of epidemics of meningococcus meningitis that occurred with the onset of barrack life in the U.S. Army (p. 193).

Most pertinent of all is their summary of Hinkle and Wolff's widely known study of one hundred Chinese expatriates in New York, all of whom "had shared a life in which they had all been exposed to a rap:dly changing culture, repeated disruptions of old social patterns, and many physical dislocations." With detailed information on health histories, Hinkle and Wolff were able to distinguish between those who were consistently healthy and those who were, with a substantial degree of consistency, ill. Wolf and Goodell summarize their findings: "The healthiest members of this group are people who are able to tolerate with some ease such recurrent disruptions of their life patterns, partly because they regard such changes and disruptions as a normal and expected part of a life pattern. . . . Hinkle and Wolff infer that ill health . . . appears to occur when an individual exists in a life situation which places demands upon him that are excessive in terms of his ability to meet them" (pp. 204–205).

Finally, Kirtz and Moos (1974), in a review of the dimensions of the social environment, found links between certain health outcomes and those social environments that ranked high or low in potential for close relationships with others. Reviewing studies of growth retardation, susceptibility of disease in infants, hypertension, peptic ulcer, rheumatoid arthritis, coronary heart disease, and deaths among older persons, Kirtz and Moos found that environments that are low in potential for social relationships among people have definite, significant effects that increase both morbidity and mortality.

Thus, we see that in the second half of the twentieth century, the old belief that a specific cause exists for a specific disease has given way to the concept of multicausality. Our journey toward definitions of health and disease has shown, first, that the health-disease dichotomy is an overly simple view of health as the absence of disease and, second, that the public health perspective, although more encompassing by emphasizing the prevention of disease, is also limited in its dichotomous definition of health. That definition, with its disease-specific hypothesis, fails adequately to take into account the influence of the environment. Susser's three coordinate systems and Antonovsky's ease-disease continuum do provide a view of health that makes it possible to study the effects of many causes on an individual's state of health. However, the continuum model, despite its recognition of the multicausality of disease, fails to provide a model of the interaction of multiple causes within and without the individual.

The Systems View of Health

You may, at this point in your reading, be somewhat surprised at the complexity of the problems involved in putting together a useful definition of health and illness. Our next step is to find a conceptual framework large enough to permit us to fit together the pieces of the "what is health" puzzle. We propose the systems approach to health as the framework we need.

The word *system* has a quite ordinary meaning to us in our daily lives. Suppose you prepare to go to work or school in the morning. This action immediately puts you into the school or work system. The school system consists of two major components: transportation (to and from school) and school itself. Each of these subsystems has a number of components. Transportation, for example, involves maintaining and policing the streets and budgeting for personnel, equipment, and so forth. Likewise, the operation of the school itself involves several components: teachers, administrators, books, buildings. Your trip to school, surprisingly, takes you into a rather large system with many interconnections. We humans have created systems that function to serve our needs and desires.

More formally defined, a system is a set of any two interrelated elements or components of any kind. Systems have the following properties:

1. The behavior of any component affects the whole system. For example, in our school system model, if the teachers are not present, the system cannot function.

2. The behavior of any component is dependent on at least one other component. If the public works department has no budget to clear the roads after a snowstorm, the transportation of students to school is affected.

3. Components are interdependent with respect to one another. Students are interdependent with respect to teachers, and both are interdependent on the school system as a whole.
4. The system is more than the sum of its parts. For example, the school system functions to provide education; no single component can accomplish this.

Just as the school system provides the function of educating an individual, the health system provides the function of maintaining the individual's health. We can conceptualize the health system of an individual as being composed of three components, or subsystems—organic, social, and personal—each of which has its own elements. The organic subsystem is composed of the body regions, organs, tissues, and cells. The social subsystem is composed of a person's culture, society, community, and family. The personal subsystem is composed of an individual's thoughts, feelings, and behaviors, with regard to his or her body, mental state, and social interaction. We will call these three elements of the personal subsystem somatic, psychic, and social responsiveness.

The three major subsystems interact to maintain an individual's health, or to produce disease. When they are in balance—a state that we will call homeostasis—health is maintained; when this balance is disrupted and lost, disease is the result. The maintenance of homeostasis depends on a person's capacity to cope with or adapt to the disruptions. This capacity is affected both by the lifestyle the individual has learned and by organic factors that may be genetically determined. Genetic factors aid in resistance or susceptibility to disease of organ tissues and cells.

For example, lifestyle factors may result in the individual's perceiving the disruption and successfully adapting or may lead the individual to apply coping strategies that will bring relief from stress. In either case homeostasis and health is maintained. These factors may, however, fail to bring about an adaptation and instead either predispose the individual to a pathological process or exacerbate an already existing pathological process. The person may then develop symptoms and assume a sick role.

The health system is arranged in hierarchical order, with the social subsystem at the top and the organic subsystem at the bottom. Disruptions originate in the social subsystem and spread both downward and upward through the system. An individual subjectively experiences disruption as social stress, psychic stress or somatic stress. Social stress is experienced as group panic—a sense of panic that the individual is no longer accepted by his or her primary group, accompanied by a feeling that the individual has failed to live according to society's norms and values. Psychic stress is experienced as anxiety—a feeling of tension and, in more extreme states, of butterflies in the stomach, accompanied by shallow breathing and

Figure 2.1 *The Downward Spread of a Disruption*
(Stress-Related Psychosomatic Illness in an Unemployed Public School Teacher)

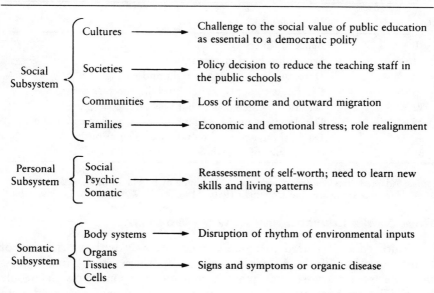

Social Subsystem	Cultures ⟶	Challenge to the social value of public education as essential to a democratic polity
	Societies ⟶	Policy decision to reduce the teaching staff in the public schools
	Communities ⟶	Loss of income and outward migration
	Families ⟶	Economic and emotional stress; role realignment
Personal Subsystem	Social Psychic Somatic ⟶	Reassessment of self-worth; need to learn new skills and living patterns
Somatic Subsystem	Body systems ⟶ Organs Tissues ⟶ Cells	Disruption of rhythm of environmental inputs Signs and symptoms or organic disease

Source: Adapted from H. L. Blum, "From a Concept of Health to a National Health Policy," *American Journal of Health Planning,* No. 1 (July 1976).

sweaty palms. Somatic stress is experienced subjectively as somatic tensions—pain and symptoms of physiologic discomfort.

Figure 2.1 presents the example of a disruption experienced by a public school teacher, which begins with a change in cultural beliefs concerning the social value of public education. The table shows the resulting stress on the individual of unemployment and the downward spread of the disruption throughout the whole system. The individual is unable to regain homeostasis, develops symptoms, and assumes a sick role.

The disruption presented in Figure 2.1 has its roots in a change in cultural beliefs—a force over which the sufferer has no direct control. There are also potential disruptions inherent in normal growth and development. Erik Erikson has charted eight developmental tasks all persons must master during their life cycle (see Table 2.2, p. 38). The tasks occur at the ages presented in the table. Failure to master a task may result in a disruption to peoples' health systems and can endanger their health. Successful mastery of a developmental task strengthens our capacity to adapt and our coping strategies both to respond to disruptions and to master future developmental tasks.

Table 2.2   *Erikson's Eight Stages of Man*

Age of Occurrence	Developmental Task
0 – 1	Belief in others
1 – 3	Separation from maternal figure
3 – 5	Development of sense of right and wrong
5 – 12	Readiness to apply oneself to skills and tasks
12 – 18	Selection of life goals (what you care to do)
18 – 30	Development of close relationships (who you care to be with)
30 – 60	Establishing and guiding the next generation
60 –	Acceptance of the wholeness of one's life

Source: Adapted from *Childhood and Society,* 2d edition by Erik H. Erikson, by permission of W. W. Norton & Company, Inc. Copyright 1950, ©1963 by W. W. Norton & Company, Inc.

How Do We Educate, and How Do We Learn?

Health educators need to be concerned not only with a definition of health but also with the meaning of education. There are two major questions we must address. First, what is education? Second, how do people learn? Throughout history, wise men and women have struggled with both questions; in neither case do we claim to have a definitive answer.

Until the Renaissance, the aim of education in Western civilization remained to mold the good man and the good citizen for the service of the state (or, especially in medieval times, for the service of God). Then, during the Renaissance, the rise of secular humanism in Europe brought with it the concept of a liberal education, the direct and overt objective of which was the liberation of the intellect from ignorance and cultivation of the mind as an instrument for critical thought. This notion of freedom of choice, based on a sophisticated method of inquiry, has become our basis for definition of the educated individual.

These two broad educational perspectives, one pre-Renaissance and the other post-Renaissance, remain very much alive in their modern contexts. We will see that theories about how people learn are based on whether individuals are to be molded to fit some preconceived conception or allowed to develop as free individuals. Each has its contemporary champion, the former belief in B. F. Skinner in his book *Walden Two* (1948) and its further justification, *Beyond Freedom and Dignity* (1975), and the latter view in A. S. Neill, in his book *Summerhill: A Radical Approach to Child Rearing* (1960).

We will see both these approaches reflected in the education of people toward better health. Some health educators prefer to mold or shape people in the direction of behavioral changes that lead to an increase in health status. Others choose to follow Dorothy Nyswander's admonition to "start where the people are" (1980, p. 14). The latter group defines their educational mission as providing individuals with the opportunity to make informed choices about health behavior.

Our second question is concerned with how people learn. People change in three ways, either through learning or through maturation or a combination of both. We define *maturation* as a developmental process within which a person from time to time manifests different traits, in other words, the blueprints that are carried in the individual's genes from the time of conception. *Learning,* on the other hand, is a change in a living individual that is not brought about by genetic inheritance. It may be a change in insight, behavior, perception, motivation, or a combination of these factors. Since educators have little effective influence on maturational patterns, they focus their energy on the learning process.

Throughout history, people have learned and taught. In most life situations we take learning for granted: people, we say, learn from experience. Parents taught children, and master workmen taught apprentices. Those who taught and those who learned felt little need to understand the process. Lecture and demonstration were the time-honored teaching methods. Students were rewarded for doing well and punished when they did poorly. Teachers served as role models for future teachers, who then taught as they had been taught as youths.

Today, the development of the field of pedagogy in the twentieth century has led to the development of theories of learning that serve as guides to the process of instruction. The question is not whether a teacher has a theory of how people learn but, rather, what theory to use. Moreover, will it be effective for the setting in which the teacher practices, and will it achieve the outcomes he or she desires? In this section, we will present several theories of learning, keeping in mind that there are no final answers about how people learn and that no theory is absolutely superior to others. We believe that different theories of learning are applicable to different situations. The competent health educator is able to both assess the learner and the learning situation and then proceed to educate on the basis of an effective and appropriate theory of instruction. The two most prominent families of contemporary learning theory are the stimulus-response (S-R) associationist and cognitive-field theories. We will examine each in turn.

Stimulus-Response Learning Theories

Contemporary S-R associationists are primarily interested in response modification. *Response modification* refers to the fate of responses that are made to certain stimuli—whether the responses will be strengthened, weakened, or changed by subsequent events. It is in this connection that the S-R associationists make continual reference to conditioning. *Condi-*

tioning means changing a response habit, and is achieved by stimulus substitution. *Substitution* is accomplished by accompanying an adequate stimulus with a new stimulus or by response strengthening or modification. (This new stimulus or response is presented with the purpose of either strengthening or changing the original stimulus.) The S-R approach, sometimes called *behavior modification,* has been found useful in the area of patient education, where problems often result from the patient's failure to comply with a health provider's instructions or adhere to a prescribed regimen.

S-R associationists are also concerned with social learning theory. For example, Clark Hull is prominent among those S-R associationists known as the reinforcement group. Hull has identified need reduction as the reinforcer that binds the response to the stimulus (1943). If a child were conditioned to say to himself "cat" when he sees a picture of a cat, Hull would postulate that this conditioning is based on some need reduction: possibly the child wants his parents' approval but his parents withhold it unless he responds as they want him to. Two other associationists, Miller and Dollard (1950), have articulated a theory of social learning and imitation based upon the Hullian theory of learning. Their principal assumption, that human behavior is learned, is based on four fundamental principles: (1) drive, (2) cue, (3) response, and (4) reward. According to social-learning theorists, the paradigm for a learned response is as follows:

Cue → (Internal Response → Drive) → External Response → Reward

A cue is a stimulus that sets off an internal response to satisfy a drive; external behavior follows. If the behavior is socially rewarded, learning has taken place.

Miller and Dollard's major modification of Hull's theory is to provide the possibility of acquired drives that are synonymous with the social context in which they occur. For example, the cue in a television commercial linking ownership of a BMW with sexual desirability might lead to an acquired drive. The external response of wishing to own the car and the commercial's rewarding approval of this wish might exemplify a learning paradigm that also could help explain how poor health habits or unhealthy lifestyles are the result of social learning. At the same time, good health habits and healthy lifestyles can be perceived as examples of social learning. Social-learning theory is therefore an important aspect of education for health educators. Its most positive use is in understanding the learning process necessary to implement programs dealing with lifestyle change.

Cognitive Field Theory

The position of Gestalt psychology is expressed in the German word *Gestalt,* which means an organized pattern or configuration or an organized whole in contrast to its individual parts. The basic notion of Gestalt theory is that a thing cannot be understood by studying its constituent parts but only by examining it in its totality, or its *membership character*. This means that the attributes or aspects of the component parts are defined by their relationship to the whole system in which they function. Clearly, this significant concept is based on the systems approach we described earlier.

Originally designed to explain perception, Gestalt theory postulates that, as viewers, we impose on a system an organization characterized by stability, simplicity, regularity, and symmetry. By imposing this organization we see an image—a tree, a house, a dog—rather than dots, colors, and shadows. When Wolfgang Kohler, in his famous study of the learning process of chimpanzees (1925), set out to test associationist ideas about learning, he observed that his apes not only displayed an accidental kind of learning (that is, S-R learning), but they also solved problems in a way he described as "insightful." Insightful learning appeared to follow the Gestalt laws of perception, and from it, the Gestalt theories of learning emerged. Most representative of these theories is the cognitive field theory of Kurt Lewin.

A key concept in understanding cognitive field theory is *insight*. Insight occurs when people pursuing their own purposes see new ways of utilizing the elements of their environment. *Learning* connotes new insights or meanings an individual has acquired. The field theorists view learning as a purposive, explorative, innovative, and creative endeavor. Learning is not seen as the linking of one thing to another, as in S-R associationist theory. Instead, the learning process is identified with thought. It is important to recognize that insights are always the learner's own; an educator cannot give an insight to a student. If we are students, teachers may acquaint us with our own insights, but they do not actually become insights for us until we see their meaning for ourselves and adopt that meaning as our own. Morris L. Bigge (1964) gives an interesting example of how insight works. He asks the student, "What is the answer to $\sqrt{(dog)^2}$?" If you know that the answer is "dog," you have an insight into the problem. However, you may never have put the insight into words. If you know that $\sqrt{x^2} = x$ and $\sqrt{4^2} = 4$, then you can verbalize a generalized rule: "the square root of anything squared is that thing." You would be making use of your insight.

Calling his method of study "group dynamics," Lewin (1961) broadened Gestalt theory to include an interest in the motivating conditions of persons in environmental situations. In an often-cited experiment, he examined the learning of individuals placed in three different social climates: anarchic, autocratic, and democratic. Lewin's basic formula is

$$B = f(P + E)$$

in which *B*, behavior, is a function (*f*) of *P*, the psychological person, and *E*, the psychological environment. A psychological person and his or her psychological environment constitute a life space, or psychological field. The psychological field is a dynamic whole of such a nature that a change in any of its parts affects every other part. It is a totality of existing events. All psychological events, such as acting, thinking, learning, hoping, and imagining are functions of mutual relationships; together they define both person and environment in mutual interaction.

Health educators are often faced with the challenge of educating individuals to change health practices. Lewin's concepts of the psychological field, group dynamics, and action research, and his conceptualization of the process of change, have long been key concepts of health education. Perhaps his most valuable contribution to health education consists of his studies of group decisions (1953). Lewin, speaking for himself, explains the importance of these studies:

> Scientifically, the question of group decision lies at the intersection of many basic problems of group life and individual psychology. It concerns the relation of motivation to action and the effect of group setting on the individual's readiness to change or to keep certain standards. It is related to one of the fundamental problems of action-research, namely, how to change group conduct so that it will not slide back to the old level within a short time. It is in this wider setting of social processes and social management that group decision should be viewed as one means of change (p. 13).

Developing his concept of change as a three-part process, Lewin went on to state that before change can take place, the individuals who are the targets of the proposed change must be ready for the possibility of change. Their current attitudes, beliefs, and practices will need *unfreezing* before alternative attitudes, beliefs, and behaviors can be seen as possible. Once unfreezing has occurred, individuals are able to experiment with alternative attitudes and behaviors, which they may then adopt. Lewin warned, however, that unless these new attitudes are *refrozen*, individuals composing an organization or community may easily return to earlier, more familiar behavior patterns. Lewin therefore developed the concept of refreezing the change on the new level so that it becomes internalized by the individual.

Lewin also postulated that learning occurs when an individual can make an informed choice of whether or not to change an already existing behavior. The learning process that leads to an informed choice is based on Lewin's concept of unfreezing previous attitudes and creating a receptivity to new knowledge that may provide the basis for the development of new attitudes. His final step is the refreezing of new attitudes that will make the changed behavior lasting. Learning can therefore be described as a "change in behavior that lasts."

Lewin's concept of change has obvious relevance to health education practice. Smoking behavior provides a good illustration. Belief barriers that defend the smoker against change must be questioned if change is to occur. Once these belief barriers are unfrozen and the smoker has selected alternative behaviors, health educators are on firm ground to assist in refreezing the new behaviors and their supporting beliefs so that the individual will not return to the previous, smoking behavior.

Lewin's notion of refreezing new behavior is not, however, appropriate for all health education efforts. It is appropriate when health educators are certain that the new behavior will further an individual's health, but it can be harmful if they are uncertain whether the new behavior will be helpful or harmful. Minkler (1980–81) points out an example in which refreezing new behavior can be harmful: the current efforts of health professionals in many developing countries to facilitate breast feeding of infants after previously promoting bottle feeding. New evidence that in some areas of the developing world bottle feeding is associated with increased infant deaths has convinced health professionals that the change is necessary, but mothers who previously learned that bottle feeding was the correct way to feed infants resist changing back to breast feeding. Once a new behavior has been accepted, it is often difficult to change.

The Link Between Health and Education

It is our intention now to provide a working definition of health education that is consistent with the definition of health and the discussion of education just presented. First, however, we must clarify the link between health and education. Earlier in the chapter, we characterized the systems approach by saying that all problems have an environment and that systems function in such a way that a change in any component of the system affects other components of the system. We have also learned that these two aspects of the systems approach are characteristic of Lewin's cognitive-field theory of learning.

The role of liberal education, as we also mentioned earlier, is to prepare the student to make wise choices: decisions made with insight and after reflection. Relying on our study of cognitive field theory, we can say that health and education are linked together when the health educator provides the learner with the opportunity to make wise choices about the improvement of the learner's status. If, however, our problem is the improvement of health, both in individuals and the society as a whole, we must consider what we have learned from the systems approach: that all problems exist in an environment. The environment relevant to this problem, as we have seen, can be the organized social system in which humanity lives. Our learner must ask the following questions: What can be changed? What is beyond our capacity as an individual, or an aggregate of individuals, to change? Finally, what are the available resources to create a change in the system?

Systems thinkers usually discriminate between the reality that can be changed and the reality that cannot be changed, by placing a boundary between the two conditions. The components of the system can be seen as the resources available for change. In our discussion of the systems approach, for example, we referred to the school as a system with the function of education. The components (teachers, administrators, books, buildings) are resources that can be used to change the functioning of the system. How do learners who wish to make informed choices about their health apply this systems model?

To answer this question, Nancy Milo has defined the organization of the health system as it relates to the range of options available to people who want health-promoting choices (Milo, 1976). She believes that the choices people have are limited to the actual and perceived options available to them. These options reflect the available resources in their personal and social environments. Most people will make the easiest choices most of the time. Most important, the range of options available to people, as well as the ease with which they may choose certain ones over others, is typically set by "a pyramid of decisions" made by the institutions and organizations, both public and private, that affect their lives. According to Milo, "The decisions taken at higher, more powerful organizational levels set the range of options available at lower levels. This may be seen in the ways in which both federal government or multinational and large-scale corporation policies concerning food, energy, transportation, or antipollution enforcement ultimately affect not only the policy-choices of public and private bodies at state and local levels, but also the individual in his and her daily choices about diet, residence, exercise, and pace of life" (p. 438).

A final link between education and health is supplied by raising the question, Who is the learner? We suggest that the learner is always the consumer—in this case, the health education consumer. Consumers can be either individuals or groups of people. They may be an individual patient, members of a community, employees of an organization, or citizens of a national body. They are, in all cases, active participants in an educational process directed toward health improvement.

Toward an Evolving Definition of Health Education

Our working definition of health education is concerned with offering consumers an opportunity to change their health-related behaviors, with the goal of achieving a more favorable position on the health-disease continuum. Changes in health-related behaviors are based on informed decisions made with an understanding of the options supplied by an individual's environment. A decision to broaden these options by changing the environment may require the effort of a number of people who have assessed the costs and benefits of this effort to themselves and others. Because health education is concerned with change, one might further suggest that health educators manipulate behavior. We suggest instead that it is current policy at organizational and societal levels that constrains personal choices. Health education when viewed from this environmental perspective offers the possibility for enlarging the choices consumers have in order to create healthful lifestyles. We note that individuals who wish to pursue destructive health practices remain free to exercise this option as long as their actions do not negatively affect the health of others. This point of view exemplifies an ethical posture of health educators and constitutes an important distinction between their position and the prevailing position held by other public health practitioners. (In Chapter 4, we will more closely examine the ethical dilemmas faced by health educators today.)

To further clarify our definition of health education, it is necessary to distinguish between health education and health promotion, a term that has become part of the new health rhetoric and is frequently used interchangeably with health education. We define *health promotion* as any combination of health education and related organizational, political, and economic interventions designed to facilitate behavioral and environmental adaptions that will improve or protect health. Health promotion, therefore, means more than health education. It should be concerned with influences on the consumer that affect the consumer's health both positively and negatively. These influences include educational messages, media advertising, the availability of products and services, laws that affect health, and the environment in which all of these factors interact. Many of these types of interventions are imposed from above or without the understanding, and certainly without the free choice, of the individuals and groups they are supposed to affect. When the two terms *health promotion* and *health education* are used interchangeably, the distinction—that health education aims at voluntary change in behavior—is overlooked. A further distinction is that although health education can be a strategy employed by those who are interested in health promotion, it is only one of a number of strategies they may choose to employ.

Health protection also differs from health education. We define *health protection* as any combination of political and economic interventions designed to facilitate behavioral and environmental adaptions to protect health. Health protection is generally concerned with health hazards in the

work place and with the presence of toxic substances. Health education
may be one of a number of strategies used to facilitate voluntary change
in the behavior of individuals or groups to reduce the presence of health
hazards. Health protection, like health promotion, relies on many additional strategies to reach its goals.

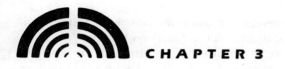

CHAPTER 3

Some Ideological Comments on Health: What Needs to Be Changed?

In Chapter 1 we traced the history of the concepts of cure and prevention from antiquity through the first and second public health revolutions and offered a role for health education in furthering prevention as a means to sound health. This challenge to health education to develop the theory and strategies necessary to change the behaviors of individuals and groups in the direction of greater health was further developed in Chapter 2, in which we offered a systems definition of health, characterized by an individual's interaction with his or her own environment, and explored the relationship between education, learning, and health education. We arrived in this chapter at an evolving definition of health education that emphasizes change in health-related behaviors among individuals and among members of organizations, communities, and societies. Before we can discuss what we mean by behavior and by change, and what educational interventions can create change in persons or groups, we must consider the environmental sources that threaten health. Then we can proceed to the question, What needs to be changed?

The Status of Health Today

Roman citizens, considered the most secure people of classical times, lived an average of little over 30 years. Life expectancy for inhabitants of Africa, Asia, and Latin America, as recently as 50 years ago, averaged only about 32 years. The decade and a half since World War II, however, saw life expectancy in the developing countries rise with a speed unequaled at any time in European and North American history.

Lay persons are likely to credit advances in modern medicine with this rapid decrease in mortality statistics. Nevertheless, health analysts have pointed out that, in spite of the effects of DDT on malaria, vaccine on the eradication of smallpox, and antibiotics on infections, modern medical technology has touched the lives of relatively few people. Rather, the dramatically upward swing in life-expectancy rates appears to be due to the equally dramatic change in general economic and social conditions. Thus, the important lifesavers have been better nutrition, improved water supplies and sanitary facilities, the spread of ideas about personal hygiene through various forms of education, and, of greatest significance, the unprecedented economic development that has raised the real wealth of billions of the world's people.

Although there continues, through the 1970's, to be a small decline in mortality figures in some wealthier countries, such as the United States, the period of quick decline seems to be at an end and, in some areas of the world, may even be reversing. A report of the World Health Organization (1975) on the status of world health stated that "after the rapid drop in mortality observed between 1950 and 1960, a 'consolidation' period is needed"; "a further decline in mortality," the report predicted, "will depend on conditions largely beyond the control of the health sector." What, we may ask, are these conditions thought to be largely beyond the control of the health sector—the unmet preconditions for good health? To help answer this question, we will briefly survey some of the causes of morbidity and mortality in both developing and developed countries. The developing countries are characterized by low per capita incomes and low technology; the developed countries are characterized by high per capita incomes and high technology.

Developing Countries

According to Sharpston (1974), in a working paper on factors determining health in developing countries, undernutrition, infections spread by human excrement, and airborne infections constitute the basic disease pattern of poverty. Although some individuals are killed directly by undernourishment, it is chronic undernutrition accompanied by infectious diseases that takes millions of lives, and takes its greatest toll among the most vulnerable members of any group: infants, children, and the aged.

Sanitary conditions usually determine the frequency with which people come into contact with infectious disease-causing agents. The World Health Organization has estimated that 1.2 billion people, or 62 percent of the inhabitants of developing countries, live without adequate water supplies. Even municipal water systems, in those areas of developing countries where water supplies are adequate, provide water of unreliable quality. Added to problems of water economy are problems of sewage treatment: raw sewage, for example, is the principal conveyor of the intestinal infections (diarrhea, cholera, and typhoid) that are the leading causes of death in those countries in which two-thirds of the world's people live.

Malaria, schistosomiasis, and filariasis are the three major diseases of the tropics; trypanosomiasis, leprosy, and leishmaniosis are the major infectious diseases that afflict the inhabitants of developing countries. Methods of control and treatment have scarcely been applied as yet to problems of tropical diseases in these countries. Medical technology alone, however, will not effectively arrest these diseases as long as hunger, inadequate sewage, and poor quality water continue to plague the populations in these areas.

Developed Countries

Infections and undernutrition have gradually receded as major killers in the developed countries. Their place has been taken by the degenerative diseases that have now become the major causes of mortality and morbidity in these countries. Taken together, coronary heart disease, heart attacks, stroke, and cancer cause two-thirds of all the deaths in North America, Europe, and the more developed countries of east Asia. We have mentioned in Chapter 1 the importance of personal behavior patterns such as smoking, dietary habits, alcoholism, and sedentary living as major contributors to premature death in developed countries. Another major contributor is the abuse or misuse of technology: the modern environmental health debacles resulting from leakage of nuclear radiation, chemical dumps, and pollution both in and out of the workplace.

The Boundaries of Change

Clearly, in both developing and developed countries, change is necessary if the health of the indigenous populations is to be maintained and improved. Although our concern is with the maintenance and promotion of health as a worldwide issue, space does not permit us to address in this book the problems in developing nations, other than a brief discussion on international settings for health education. We will, therefore, necessarily limit our remarks to the developed countries, with specific reference to the United States of America.

To this point we have discussed conditions both within the person and within the environment that adversely affect the health of individuals, whether they live in developed or underdeveloped countries. We have strongly committed ourselves to the belief that these conditions must be changed if health is to improve. We must now discuss, as health educators, the boundaries of our efforts for change. The conditions that con-

front us run the gamut from the somatic and personal systems to the
societal system. What systems shall we attempt to change? We may
choose as citizens to change the political, social, and economic systems of
the larger system, society; this is drawing the boundaries of our adversary
in the broadest possible way. What are the boundaries we need to establish for ourselves in our role as health educators? What are the boundaries
of a health system?

From the point of view of ideal change, the question of boundaries
makes little sense. For example, the boundaries of a health system cannot
simply be determined by the national boundaries of a country: poverty,
undernutrition, poor sanitation, technological abuses, and unhealthy lifestyles are not contained within national limits. Nor does the issue of
health alone bound the system, for health is strongly influenced by poverty, social conditions, and a wide range of other factors. Brown and Margo (1978) are major spokespersons in health education for this point of
view. Espousing an ecological view of health education, they believe that
health educators can develop a "work role in which as health professionals they help change social conditions that make people sick, literally."
Criticizing health educators for having lapsed into the role of "technicians
drawing plans for social change," Brown and Margo instead propose that
health educators could "provide the means for people to examine the social bases of their work and lives for unhealthful conditions and to help
give them tools to change those conditions." They note that "this is a
substantially different role than putting complete responsibility on the individual for changing unhealthful behavior, although it definitely retains a
strong emphasis on the responsibility of individuals to participate and
take the lead in alleviating such conditions" (Brown and Margo, 1978, p.
14). In such a model, the role of the health educator is to help foster the
unfolding of the change process.

Other health professionals have responded to such criticisms by stating
that Brown and Margo have defined the system too broadly and that unless the boundaries are more narrowly defined, it is impossible to effect
change. They believe that if health educators wish to offer the client an
opportunity to change health-related behavior, we must first explicitly define the boundaries of the client's system. They further suggest an approach to drawing those boundaries, using the equation we developed in
Chapter 1:

$$Hs = (f) E + AcHS + B + Ls$$

which means that the health status of an individual is a function of the
individual's environment, access to health services, biology, and lifestyle.
This equation reflects our systems approach, in which we outlined three
major subsystems—the personal, the somatic, and the social. We can now
add a fourth subsystem—the health care delivery system (*HCDS*), a neces-

sary part of the ingredient "access to health services" (*AcHS*). By offering a variety of services dealing with care, cure, and prevention, the health care delivery system ensures that individuals will receive health services in order to improve their health status. If the boundaries of the system are drawn so that health educators offer their services as part of the health care delivery system, then this system becomes the arena for the practice of health education.

We have so far drawn those boundaries to include individuals who enter the health care delivery system. Health educators, however, also provide health education to groups with the aim of changing the structure of an organization or a community when this change can improve the health status of members of these groups. We have borrowed two terms from sociology, *micro unit* and *macro unit,* to refer to change in individuals and change in groups. The health educator whose goal is to provide an educational experience for an individual or a number of individuals who wish to stop smoking has set a system boundary based on micro change. The health educator whose aim is to change practices in an organization that places its employees at risk of incurring hypertension has set a system boundary based on macro change.

The Health Care Delivery System

Having established the health care delivery system as the arena for the practice for health education, we will now examine the system more closely. In this section we will describe the current model of health care delivery, review some major critiques of the system, discuss the social values held by our society and how they influence the system, and, finally, provide a workable model of the system as we believe it should look.

The Current Model of Health Care Delivery

One way to describe the health care delivery system is to use the systems approach we developed in Chapter 2. In this systems model we need the following variables:

1. An external environment composed of a society that exerts external social forces or influences, including sociocultural, economic, technological, political, and legal forces
2. A variety of institutions within this society where people may go to obtain health services or products
3. People, with their own interests, who desire services and products of institutions, in order to pursue their goals of becoming healthy

Further, as Figure 3.1 shows (see p. 52), our model may be analyzed in terms of inputs, processes, and outputs. These categories clearly define a

Figure 3.1 *A Systems Model of Health Care Delivery*

External Constraints

Sociocultural forces
Economic forces
Technological forces
Political forces
Legal forces

Inputs: Illness

Individuals with health needs

Groups with disease

Environmental factors
contributing to disease

HEALTH CARE
DELIVERY SYSTEM

(processes involving
delivery of health care)

Outputs: Health

Individuals

Groups

Environmental factors

Health Service Points Distributed Within System

Structural Features	Setting(s)	Type(s) of Service	Level of Prevention
Facility	Hospital	Medical	Primary
Organization	Home	Social	Secondary
Finance	School	Wellness	Tertiary
Personnel	Voluntary	Nutritional	
Accountability	organization	Occupational	
	Workplace	Mental/emotional	
	Clinic	Etc.	
	Health		
	department		

Objectives

Quality
Continuity
Efficiency
Accessibility

set of variables within the system, a set of functions that measure the efficiency and effectiveness of the system, and a set of variables that are external to the health system but that have an impact upon it.

Inputs into the system are people pursuing their own interests and seeking assistance from institutions in solving their health problems. Their goal is to "become healthy." The means is through the process of interaction with a variety of institutions within society where people obtain health services or products. For example, an individual might have a disease or condition about which they can act to improve their health.

People enter the health system at many different health service points. Each point, which represents a specific site or location for the provision of health services, can be described according to four variables: (1) geographic setting (e.g., hospital, physician's office, or home), (2) type of service (medical, surgical, psychiatric, etc.), (3) level of prevention (primary, secondary, or tertiary), and (4) structural features (facility, organization, finance, personnel, and accountability). As consumers enter the health system, or move from point to point, they may encounter difficulties or barriers that slow down or ultimately block their progress toward achieving their goal of becoming healthy. These barriers can be described with a second series of variables labeled accessibility, quality, continuity, and efficiency. Finally, a third set of variables exists outside of the health system but greatly influences how it operates. These variables, referred to as external constraints, include sociocultural, economic, technological, legal, and political forces.

The model presented in Figure 3.1 serves to illustrate the variety of perspectives necessary to operationally define a health system. It clearly identifies important distinctions between the structure of the system, the processes involved as clients interact with the system, and the outcomes consumers seek. As Donabedian (1973) has made clear, "Structure signifies the properties of the resources used to provide care and the manner in which they are organized" (p. 55); as such, it involves the settings and instrumentalities available and used for the provision of health. The structural features of a health system include how it is organized and financed, who provides the services, where they are located, and who is responsible for insuring that consumers' needs are met. In contrast, "process" consists of the activities of health professionals in the management of consumers' problems or needs; it emphasizes "the degree to which the provision of service for the consumer conforms with the standards and expectations of the profession" (p. 57).

Figure 3.2 (see p. 54) is a schematic presentation of the medical care process suggested by Donabedian (1973, p. 59). It shows two parallel events, one related to the client and the other to the care provider. Generally the client enters the process in response to some need perceived as a disturbance of health or well-being. The process of seeking care and cure

Figure 3.2   *The Medical Care Process*

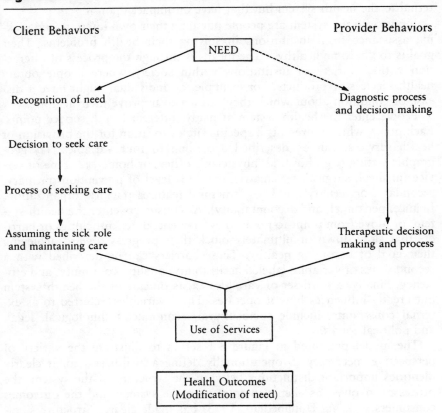

Client Behaviors   Provider Behaviors

NEED

Recognition of need   Diagnostic process
                                                   and decision making

Decision to seek care

Process of seeking care

Assuming the sick role   Therapeutic decision
and maintaining care   making and process

Use of Services

Health Outcomes
(Modification of need)

Source: Adapted from Avedis Donabedian, *Aspects of Medical Care Administration* (Cambridge, Mass.: Harvard University Press, 1973), by permission of the publisher.

leads to the provider, who initiates a parallel set of events, which includes the diagnostic process and therapeutic decision-making process. The activities of client and provider then converge in the use of a service, which should result in the alleviation of the need that set the whole process in motion.

That end result of the process of interaction with the system—the "outcome"—is usually measured in terms of the consumer's change in health status. If there is an improvement as measured by a positive change on a health scale (e.g., morbidity, mortality), then the services provided are judged "good" or "valuable" to the consumer.

We will now use our systems model to review a variety of criticisms that have been leveled at the existing health care delivery system.

Critiques of the Health Care Delivery System

We have selected three major critiques of the current health care delivery system in order to present a range of perceptions about what needs to be changed in this model. The first two, by Ivan Illich (1976) and Vincent Navarro (1976), criticize the system because it overlooks the environment in which the delivery of health care takes place. This is the inevitable weakness of a model based on a process (the delivery of medical care), which neither defines the environment nor explains how the environment shapes the process of delivery of services. The third, a feminist analysis, focuses on the failure of the health care delivery system to take into account the unique somatic, psychic, and social factors that influence women's lives, as well as the ways in which women influence the process of health service delivery. Feminist critics have drawn attention to the social values implicit in the process of health care delivery—values that they feel result in a denial of the personal freedom of women to obtain adequate care. Although the critiques of Navarro and Illich deal with what may seem to be more general concerns of self-care versus authoritarianism, mystification, and "medicalization," feminists have correctly pointed out that women's issues cannot be separated from those concerned with the general welfare.

Illich's Critique.   Illich (1976) uses the term *iatrogenic* to describe the current health care delivery system. The dictionary defines *iatrogenic* as referring to an illness caused by what a healer does or prescribes. Illich finds medical care iatrogenic in three different ways. First are the "undesirable side effects of approved, mistaken, callous, or contra-indicated technical contacts with the system" (p. 32); second, the effects of a medical practice that "sponsors sickness by reinforcing a morbid society that encourages people to become consumers of curative, preventative, industrial, and environmental medicine" (p. 33); and, third, the "even deeper, culturally health-denying effects" of the "so-called health professions" as they "destroy the potential of people to deal with their human weakness, vulnerability, and uniqueness" (p. 33). Illich, therefore, sees professionalization as having "medicalized" society to the point at which it robs people of their health by creating a situation in which they feel unable to rely on themselves to cope with their environment, their bodies, and their illness.

Navarro's Critique.   Basing his analysis on contemporary Marxist ideology, Navarro (1976) charges that the growing socialization of production leads inevitably to greater state intervention in order to ensure continued accumulation of private capital and profit. The growth of state intervention and expense leads to a continuous crisis of budget deficits and, thus, in the need to increase taxes, which in turn are forever insufficient for making up the deficits. The state's response to this crisis has been and continues to be cutting social programs, further centralization of state power, and higher productivity of both workers and capital. The effect of the system leads to cuts in health expenditures, especially for the under-served populations—the elderly, welfare recipients, children, and minorities. These cuts are rationalized by a cost-benefit analysis in which the argument is put forth that, since these groups contribute least to the productivity of the system, the costs of providing them with adequate health care far outweigh the benefits to the system.

The Feminist Critique. Feminists have offered a third critique of the health care delivery system that is of growing importance to the field of health care and the goals and objectives of health education. Beginning their analysis with the premise of the right of women to maintain control over their own bodies, feminists have argued that in early recorded history the process of reproduction was essentially under the control of women but that it later came to be "medicalized" by a male-dominated medical profession, with the consequence that pregnancy was defined as an illness to be managed by health professionals. With the spread of Western medicine, these and other harmful beliefs have spread throughout much of the world. According to the Boston Women's Health Collective (1980), "as modern, Western-based medicine becomes an integral part of 'development' programs, indigenous systems of belief and care are destroyed or actively persecuted by medical 'authorities.' This is especially ironic since modern medicine itself is becoming only more costly and less accessible to people almost everywhere. Women, especially, have suffered from the expansion of modern medical institutions" (p. 14).

Feminists believe that decision-making opportunities for women must be provided at the individual and policy-making levels. The policy-making level includes proposals to determine what ought to be the policies of hospitals, medical professional associations, pharmaceutical companies, and federal regulatory agencies about how women, as clients, will be treated. Holmes and Peterson (1981) point out that these policy-making issues involve careful study of ethical dilemmas. According to the feminist argument, most current discussions of ethical dilemmas are based on a patriarchal definition of rights that is fundamentally adversarial and negative. A feminist view of rights, in contrast, emphasizes positive values such as helpfulness, cooperation, and relatedness. Thus, the right over one's body advocated by feminists raises ethical issues not raised by traditional ethical scholarship.

Basic Values Relevant to Health Care

The three critiques that we have briefly summarized each point out that the current health care delivery system is not functioning effectively to provide cure, care, or prevention. In order realistically to present a design of a system that will meet some of the objections we have reviewed, we must first look at the basic social values that affect our perception of what health care delivery should be and do.

As Donabedian (1973) makes clear in his discussion of social values and health care,

> Social values permeate a society and all of its institutions. To a considerable degree such values are responsible for the forms that these institutions take and the directions along which they may be acceptably modified. The institutionalized forms for the provision of health services are no exception to this rule. Social values may, in fact, be more than usually relevant. This is because medical care touches upon the most vital concerns of people, involves intimate and intensely personal relationships, and is surrounded by a variety of moral and ethical prescriptions (p. 14).

Although the relationship of social values to health services may seem so simple as to be self-evident, we consider it important for three reasons. The first of these is that in a democratic society, citizens vote for parties and individuals whose avowed policies are based on these values. The second reason is that because these values are largely implicit, their influence on behavior may escape notice. A third reason rests upon the fact that social values are acquired through the process of socialization, usually beginning in childhood, with the result that they are accepted and strongly defended when challenged. It is our purpose to make explicit those values that we believe are implicit to the health care system.

Donabedian refers to four social values basic to the health care system. These are personal responsibility, social concern, freedom, and equality. Although individuals may express a variety of attitudes about each of these social values, we can identify two major positions or viewpoints with respect to health issues. We will, in accordance with American political terminology, refer to one viewpoint as *libertarian* and the other as *egalitarian*. The libertarian viewpoint places major emphasis on personal achievement and the freedom of the individual. The egalitarian position is primarily concerned with equality of opportunity and perceives freedom as the key to equalizing opportunities for choice.

A case in point would be the differing positions on national health insurance taken by the libertarians, usually represented by Republican presidential administrations, and the egalitarians, who generally find their place in Democratic administrations. The libertarian position is that people should assume personal responsibility for their health care. They express their social concern by their belief that the government should leave the business of providing health service to the private sector, which they state is better equipped to provide both quality and cost-effective health care. They further believe that if the government makes provision for health care, it infringes on the freedom of individuals to select their own kind of services and on the freedom of the health profession to deliver those services in the most efficient manner. Finally, they interpret equality as meaning that all individuals should have an equal opportunity to enter the marketplace and compete for health services.

The egalitarian position holds that all individuals are members of their community and citizens of the state. This membership includes a responsibility of all for all; each of us is responsible to see that health services are available to our fellow citizens. Community members can discharge this responsibility through their government, which then assumes the responsibility for health services for all citizens through the passage of a national health insurance act. Egalitarians have, along with this sense of personal responsibility, a social concern that their responsibility be directed toward and translated into actions that benefit humankind. A national health insurance act would exemplify the translation of their social concern into action. Moreover, such an act would be consistent with the egalitarian notion of freedom as providing opportunities for all individuals to have equal access to health care. By providing public financing for health care, national health insurance would assure the needy equal opportunity with all others to be recipients of health care. Finally, egalitarians view freedom as the freedom to act that occurs when all people share the same options. In the case of health care, all individuals served under national health insurance would be free to apply for health services without the limitation imposed by their ability to pay for services.

As one point of view, we have presented the idea that personal beliefs strongly color designs of programs and recommendations for action in the health care field. This book necessarily reflects the personal beliefs of the authors; as a reader, you should know where we stand so that you can better evaluate the material we have presented. It has, possibly, become clear by this chapter that we subscribe to the egalitarian viewpoint. It is from this position that we state our belief that requirements for a health care delivery system include allowances for individual choice, equitable access, and a systems approach to individual health and health care.

Furthermore, we believe that deficient health care is not the major cause of poor health status in the United States. Rather, the major determinants of poor health are unsatisfactory living conditions associated with urban overcrowding, poverty, minority status, inadequate and unsafe transportation, and unhealthful lifestyles that have developed as ways of coping with these conditions of life. We further believe that all persons must have access to comprehensive prepaid delivery systems. There should be public financing to support health care delivery systems so that consumers face no obstacle to care and providers are ensured adequate compensation. Finally, since the problems of prevention and care are interrelated, they must be addressed simultaneously. We can now turn our attention to a proposed design of the health care delivery system and those functions we believe it should serve.

The Health Care Delivery System: A Proposed Model

In Chapter 2 we developed a conceptual model of health based on systems theory. We then proceeded to characterize the forces that affect health—on the societal, personal, and somatic levels—and described our personal position on social values. Our task now is to expand our proposed model of the health care delivery system. The model, in keeping with our egalitarian position on social values, provides for individual choice and equitable access to the system, and reflects a systems approach to health care.

A health care delivery system that is concerned with care, cure, and health promotion must serve three diverse functions. First, it must provide services that are relevant to persons expressing a complaint about a problem or a hurt that affects their somatic, psychic, or social health. Second, it must provide services that offer individuals opportunities to change attitudes and behaviors related to those aspects of one's life over which one has some control. Third, the system must promote "survival wisdom" by involving its subscribers both in its own activities and in the activities of society at large. This involvement would be expected to both inform subscribers and to motivate them to bring about changes in the large environmental forces that directly affect their health. Examples of these forces include unemployment; discrimination; unsafe housing; excessive speed limits; air, water, soil, and food pollution; and dangerous work environments.

Figure 3.3 (see p. 60) represents a health care delivery system that emphasizes a primary well-being center with related, increasingly specialized secondary and tertiary centers (Blum, 1976). The medical care delivery system is one component of the system. Others are social support services, social control services, and psychic support and control services. The primary well-being center is the unit of delivery of health care; the secondary and tertiary centers are subunits. The two-way arrows indicate that the primary, secondary, and tertiary units of each subsystem are heavily interconnected. We should note that unlike Figure 3.2, which represents a model of a process, Figure 3.3 presents a structural model. This is because a system can best be expressed as a structure composed of parts or components that are interrelated. The interrelationship in this model is between the somatic, social, and psychic services components and between each service and the primary, secondary, and tertiary centers of that service.

Because Blum envisions the primary well-being center as the basic unit of a health care delivery system, the primary attributes of the center are of

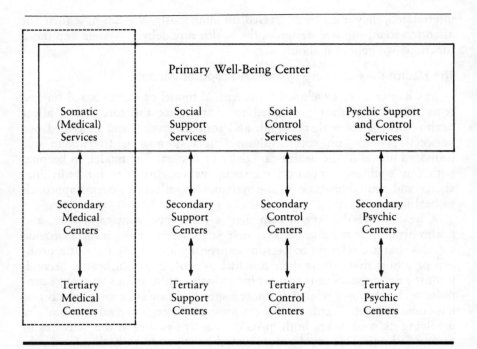

Figure 3.3   *The Primary Well-Being Center
(in a Structural Model of the Health Care Delivery System)*

Source: Adapted from H. L. Blum, "From a Concept of Health to a National Health Policy,"
American Journal of Health Planning, No. 1 (July 1976).

significant interest to health educators. These micro-level attributes include (1) providing possibilities of new health behaviors to individuals
who are being treated for illness; (2) strengthening health and reducing
risks of illness by offering all members programs to provide learning
about behaviors; (3) offering all subscribers a model of health-promotive
and health-preserving behaviors; (4) offering programs that give members
the opportunity to see the effects of their own behaviors on their health
status; and (5) making educational opportunities available to people in
situations that place them at risk and teaching them how to cope with
these situations.

Some macro-level attributes of the well-being center include providing
subscribers with opportunities (1) to learn about issues relating to health,
ecology, and their physical environment; (2) providing members with educational opportunities about issues of health care and their relationship to
socioeconomic disruptions, such as unemployment, crime, addiction, war;
and (3) offering members opportunities for involvement in community ef-

forts related to health (i.e., regional and statewide health planning, the economy, ecology, environmental housing, employment) and in community activities related to decisions about the allocation of public resources in such areas as housing, transportation, education, and health.

The most significant challenge that faces health educators today is the need to help change national health policy so that current health care delivery systems reflect the criteria and attributes just enumerated. A truly egalitarian national health policy would set priorities, first, to provide adequate funding for a wide range of projects devoted to the improvement of the nation's health, including rehabilitation of the country's urban centers, creation of reliable mass transit systems, and reduction of poverty. Funding for these projects would be separate from additional moneys set aside to support the nation's health care through development of health care delivery systems based on well-being centers as the primary unit of delivery. A second priority is to ensure that the services of at least one health care delivery system are available to every person in the United States. As a third priority, these systems should be locally governed by consumer-dominated groups.

It is not our intention to provide a blueprint for a national health policy. Instead, we hope to give the reader an opportunity to observe the direction in which we believe change can and should be directed. We have, by offering this information, come full circle from the beginning of this chapter, where we discussed what needs to be changed, to the end, where we have suggested a model and a direction for change in the health care sector of society.

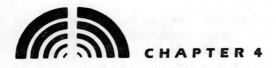

CHAPTER 4

How, and for Whom, Health Educators Create Change

We have thus far established a working definition of health education which states that health education is concerned with offering consumers opportunities to change their health-related behaviors, with the goal of achieving a more favorable position on the health-disease continuum. We are now ready to explore how, and for whom, health educators create change. To enhance the clear exposition of this topic, Chapter 4 has been divided into several sections, in which we will examine (1) change from a theoretical and practical perspective, (2) educational interventions that create behavioral changes and how these educational strategies work with individuals and groups in organizations and communities, (3) an evolving theory of behavioral and social change, (4) the effects of social values on health educators' efforts for change, and (5) the ethical dilemmas that arise when one acts to change the behavior of others.

Understanding Change

A Theoretical Perspective

Before we can examine how to foster behavioral changes, we need first to arrive at a suitable definition of behavior. Let us say that *behavior* consists of those activities of a human being, or any other organism, that can be observed directly or by means of specialized instruments or techniques. Thus, walking and speaking are forms of behavior. There are, however, less easily observed forms. For example, although a person charged with a crime may appear calm and show no easily detectable behavior, a psychologist using special instruments may be able to detect this behavior in the individual's changes in blood pressure, breathing, and pulse rate. Methods also exist for detecting and measuring less tangible forms of behavior, such as learning and reasoning.

In addition to our definition of behavior, two other concepts are important to achieving a theoretical understanding of behavior change. These are the concepts of first-order change and second-order change. *First-order change* occurs within a group. We will show by examples that once individuals have been identified as being members of a specific class or group (e.g., students), they can undergo very limited changes in behavior while they are functioning as members of that group. Thus, students will behave as students. *Second-order change* is initiated from outside the group—that is, by someone who is not bound by the rules of group membership and can, therefore, more easily suggest significant changes in the behavior of group members. These changes provide group members with opportunities to solve problems that were previously seen by them as insoluble.

There are few of us who have not wondered why we persist in behaviors that we would like to change. Many smokers are well aware, for example, that smoking is hazardous to their health, but in spite of their wish to stop, all too few of them are able to change their behavior. (The persistence of unhealthy behaviors holds true as well in the areas of diet, exercise, and exposure to stress.) Furthermore, who has not wanted to change organizational behavior—for example, when we chafe under restrictions that define our behavior at work in ways that conflict with much that we have learned in preparation for our careers. Individuals employed in both helping and health professions recall that when they were in school preparing for their professions, they were admonished that the clients' needs and health were to be their paramount concern. Yet teachers, nurses, and health educators frequently speak of the conflict between the needs of the organization for which they work and the needs of the clients they have been trained to serve. Teachers wonder why they must act as disciplinarians, a role frequently in conflict with that of educator; nurses have come to believe that they must uphold the rules of the hospital, even when those rules lead to poor and inadequate patient care. Similarly, health educators are assigned to implement program plans for stress reduction in individuals who work in environments that are inherently stressful, knowing they are not allowed to help change the stressful environment.

These concerns about behavior on both the personal and organizational levels lead us to wonder why behaviors persist in spite of our stated wish to change them. We also are concerned with what is required to bring about the changes we wish to take place.

Change Within a System.　Watzlawick (1974) has given us some interesting theoretical ways to think about these questions. First, he asks us to look at the theory of the properties of groups as developed by the great French mathematician Evariste Galois. Group theory gives us a framework for understanding the kind of change that can occur within a system. It requires only a moment's thought to see that "grouping" or "ordering" things is basic to our sense of perception and our way of knowing reality. Although no two things can ever be exactly similar, by ordering things that share an important property in common, we give structure and meaning to our world. Watzlawick points out that, according to Galois's conception of group theory, a group can be described in terms of four properties. First,

> A) It (a group) is composed of members which are all alike in one common characteristic, while their actual nature is otherwise irrelevant for the purposes of the theory. They can thus be numbers, objects, concepts, events, or whatever else one wants to draw together in such a group, as long as they have that common denominator and as long as the outcome of any combination of two or more members is itself a member of the group (p. 3).

If we establish, for example, that the six animals in Figure 4.1 are members of a group because of their common characteristic (all are foxes), then any combination of two or more foxes will also be a member of the group of foxes. (In Galois's definition, "combination" refers to the addition or subtraction of members; thus, if we subtract two foxes from five foxes, the result, three foxes, still constitutes a part of the group.) The grouping of things is a universal means by which we can make sense out of reality even though no two things are exactly alike (our foxes may differ slightly in height and weight); thus, the ordering of the world into groups composed of members that all share an important element in common gives structure to a world that would otherwise be chaos.

Once we have established a group based on something all members have in common, like foxiness, it becomes impossible for any member or combination of members to place themselves outside of the group. A fox is a fox, and two or more foxes are still members of the group *fox*. As Watzlawick explains,

> B) Another property of a group is one that may combine its members in varying sequence, yet the outcome of the combination remains the same. A practical example would be this: Starting from a given point on a surface and making any number of moves of any individual length and direction, one invariably and inevitably reaches the same destination, regardless of any change in the sequence of moves—provided, of course, that the number of these moves as well as their individual length and direction remain the same (p. 4).

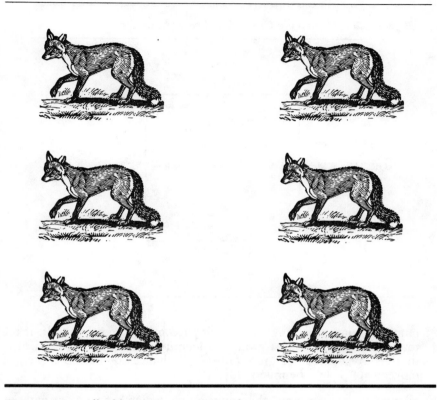

Figure 4.1   *All Alike in One Common Characteristic: Foxes*

For instance, in the example in Figure 4.2 (see p. 66) we have four moves, each made in the direction of each of the cardinal points of the compass and each of the same unit of distance (e.g., one inch or one mile). We start east, then go south, then west, and finally north, ending where we had begun our travel. Regardless of the sequence (first east, then south, or whatever sequence you choose), we are always back at the starting point at the completion of the fourth move. From this example, we might conclude that there is changeability in process—in this case directional change—but no change in outcome.

According to Watzlawick's third property,

C) A group contains an identity number such that its combination with any other member defines that other member, which means that it maintains that other member's identity. For instance, in groups whose rule of combination is additive, the identity number is zero (e.g., $5 + 0 = 5$); in groups whose combination rule is multiplication, the identity

Figure 4.2   *Combining Group Members in Sequence*

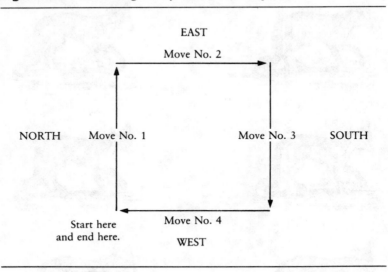

number is one, since any entity multiplied by one remains itself. If the total of all sounds was a group, its identity number would be silence, the identity number of the group of all changes of positions (i.e., of movements) would be immobility.

In relation to our concerns, the point is that a member may act without making a difference.

And finally, the fourth property:

D) ... in any system satisfying the group concept, we find that every member has its reciprocal or opposite. In other words, the combination of any member, with its opposite, gives the identity member; (e.g., where the combination rule is addition, $5 + (-5) = 0$). Again, we see that on one hand this combination produces a marked change, but on the other hand, the result is itself a member of the group (in the present example the positive and negative integers, including zero) and is thus contained within it (p. 5).

Assume, for example, that Harry and Tom are members of a group, and that Harry has just lost two dollars to Tom. First, Harry had two dollars and Tom had nothing; now Harry is minus two dollars and Tom has two dollars while Harry has nothing. The equation for Harry and Tom's transaction is $\$2 + (-\$2) = 0$. Although a shift of funds has occurred between the two group members, the group has not become richer or poorer. The system itself has not changed.

Group theory gives us a way of thinking about the kinds of change that can occur within a group or system that itself does not change. We believe this conceptualization is helpful in clarifying problems of change, whether within an individual or an institution. We will use Watzlawick's term "first-order change" to refer to this kind of change.

Change from Outside a System.   Another theory concerned with change, the theory of logical types, explains the relationship between the *class* (a group whose members are all alike in that they share a common characteristic) and the process by which the class shifts to a higher logical level. Watzlawick (1974) again will be our guide. Using the example of a person having a nightmare, he illustrates a second kind of change, different from that described in group theory:

> The sleeper can do many things in his dream, he can run or hide, fight or yell. None of these changes, however, would ever end the dream. There is only one way out of the nightmare and that is for the dreamer to waken. The change from dreaming to waking means, of course, that the dreamer is no longer asleep. Therefore, the dream is a change to a different state of consciousness (p. 10).

Watzlawick refers to this kind of a change as a "change of a change" and has named it "second-order change."

If we look back to the preceding section at Galois's group theory, we observe that the four properties of any group responsible for creating change within the group (combination, sequence, identity, and reciprocity) are not themselves members of the group. According to Watzlawick, "This becomes particularly evident with reference to the combination rules holding for a particular group":

> We saw, for instance, that where the internal group operations are effected by the rule of multiplication, the identity number is one.
>
> If the combination rule in this group was changed to addition (a second-order change that could only be introduced from the outside and could not be generated from within the group), there would be a different outcome: member n combined with the identity number (1) would no longer be itself (as it would be under the old rule, where n multiplied by one would again give n), but we would obtain $n + 1$.

Watzlawick concludes that these effects of changing the combination rule mean that "groups are invariant only on the first-order change level (i.e., on the level of change from one member to another, where, indeed, the more things change, the more they remain the same), but are open to change on the second-order change level (i.e., to changes in the body of rules governing their structure or internal order." In sum, group theory and the theory of logical types "thus reveal themselves not only as compatible with each other, but also complementary" (p. 122).

Some Practical Examples Illustrating First- and Second-Order Change

The preceding section established a distinction between first- and second-order change in theoretical terms. We will now illustrate this distinction as it applies to real-life situations.

In group theory, the first group property, A (any combination, transformation, or operation on group member gives a group member), functions to maintain group structure. Consider this example from occupational health. The management of a large hospital has traditionally been responsible for employee health and safety at the workplace. When a recent study by an outside consulting firm documents that the hospital has had a poor safety record and recommends shifting the responsibility for health and safety to a committee composed of both employees and management, the resulting change is a new combination of members but no basic change in the hospital's group structure, as far as health and safety are concerned.

Group property B is concerned with the idea that a sequence of operations (performed on group members in accordance with the combination rule for that group) may be changed without changing the result of the operations themselves. The result is a change in process but not in outcome. We can see this concept exemplified by problem drinkers who provoke their spouses to criticize their drinking behavior. The more the spouse complains, the more the drinking increases. The more the drinking increases, the more the spouse implores the drinker to stop. What is significant is that the spouse comments on the drinking: it does not matter whether the comments are for or against. Neither acceptance nor rejection will cause the drinker to stop. In other words, the process may be affected but the outcome will not change.

The third group property, C, states that a group contains an identity number that in combination with any one member gives that member. (Remember our example that $5 + 0 = 5$, where 0 is the identity number.) This means that the number acquires stability. The importance of the concept of stability in this instance is that a member may act without effecting any change. From a practical point of view, a society's traditions can be seen as having the function of an identity number. For example, in the campaign against abortion by the group called the Moral Majority, the Bible is cited as evidence that abortion runs counter to Christian belief. After thus establishing that having abortions is bad, the Moral Majority then propose to force people not to have abortions. The ultimate result would not be to eliminate abortions, as the group proposes, but to create an underground movement. People not only will continue to get abortions but will do so at the risk of criminal prosecution.

Group property D deals with the replacement of something with its opposite—which appears to be a significant change, since it is based on the false belief that if something is bad, its opposite must be good. For example, the strong interest in self-care in the health field rests on the belief that the dependency of people on the health care establishment is both harmful and expensive. People must care for themselves! Self-care, however, does not affect individuals' underlying dependencies on the unhealthy practices of the society in which they live. A more personal example involves the woman who divorces a domineering man in order to marry a sensitive, supportive husband, only to discover that, whereas she expected the second marriage to be the opposite of the first, nothing has changed. Her quiet spouse seems to restrict her freedom in the marriage in quiet ways, as her previous husband had through active domination.

Our examples of change in relation to these four group properties clarify both the limits of first-order change and the built-in resistance of any system to it. Consequently, to achieve second-order change we must step outside the system. This distinction between inside and outside may best be explained by one of the basic tenets of anthropology: that it is very difficult to arrive at more than a superficial understanding of one's own culture until one has left it. Accordingly, one must be prepared for a shock when one's own culture is seen from the vantage point of another culture.

Watzlawick (1974) gives a simple illustration of the need to go outside the system in solving problems whose solutions are not contained in the internal rules governing the system. The nine dots in Figure 4.3 (p. 70) can be connected by four straight lines without lifting the pencil from the paper. (We suggest that the reader who is not familiar with this problem try to find the solution on a separate piece of paper before reading on and especially before turning to the solution.) Almost everyone who tries to solve this problem initially goes astray by relying on an assumption that makes the solution impossible to obtain. The assumption—that the dots compose a square and that the solution must be found within that square —is a self-imposed condition that the instructions do not contain. Failure, therefore, does not lie in the impossibility of the task, but in the method of arriving at a solution. Having now created the problem, we discover that it does not matter which combination of four lines is tried, or in what order. There will always be at least one unconnected dot. In other words, we can run through the totality of the first-order change possibilities existing within the square, but will never solve the task. The solution is a second-order change, which consists in leaving the field.

Very few people are able to solve the nine-dot problem without first understanding this concept. Those who fail and give up are usually surprised at the unexpected simplicity of the solution (see Figure 4.4, p. 72).

The nine-dot problem demonstrates that second-order change is a simple change from one set of premises to another set of the same logical type. The first set assumes that in order to solve the task you must keep

---

Figure 4.3 *The Nine-Dot Problem*

Connect the nine dots with four straight lines, without
lifting the pencil from the paper.

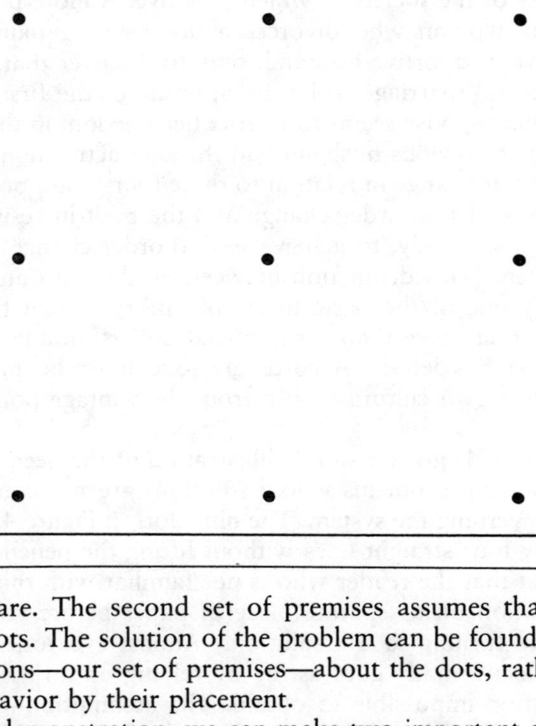

•   •   •

•   •   •

•   •   •

---

within a square. The second set of premises assumes that you may go
beyond the dots. The solution of the problem can be found if we examine
our assumptions—our set of premises—about the dots, rather than determine our behavior by their placement.

From this demonstration, we can make two important generalizations.
The first is that the theory of logical types makes it clear we must not talk
about a class or group in language appropriate for its members. (In Figures 4.3 and 4.4 the members are the dots; the whole configuration is the
class or group.) The second generalization is that we must recognize that
the rules are real only to the extent to which we have created them. Therefore, we are free to change the rules (our set of premises) if we wish.

We can make immediate practical application of our theories of first-
and second-order change by using them to understand the differences between health educators who are primarily involved in patient education
through behavior modification and health educators who envision and are
involved in lifestyle change. The former usually work toward first-order
change—change from one behavior to another within a given way of behaving. In contrast, lifestyle change is primarily concerned with second-
order change—change from one way of behaving to another.

Understanding Educational Interventions

Human behavior tends toward stability; it tends to persist. Another way of describing persistence is to argue that all human behavior—individual, group, organizational, and societal—tends to be cyclical in nature. Individuals engage in much the same behavior within a given time frame and within given settings. That is, we generally organize our activities on the basis of an established routine. Problematic aspects of this form of behavior are exhibited, for example, by smokers who start off with their first cigarette after breakfast, have the next one during morning break, and so on throughout the day. Although these smokers promise themselves and others that "this is the last one," they continue to follow this pattern day after day, against their stated wishes.

Groups behave in much the same way. Family disagreements seem to be played out in a repetitive, predictable fashion with various family members sticking to their roles of the good guy, the negotiator, the troublemaker, and so on. Organizations surely have their cyclical or persistent behaviors; indeed, the term *bureaucracy* has lost much of its original meaning of institutional organization for efficient task performance and has come, instead, to connote persistent problematical and often ineffective behavior.

Societies also behave in stable, cyclical patterns. U.S. political and military leaders are currently at consensus, stating that we must stay ahead in the armaments race. Both U.S. and Soviet leaders strike this posture, with the probable result that if the armaments race continues, it will be at great cost and sacrifice to millions. Neither side publicly addresses the question of what happens when we achieve a state of mutual deterrence. Can we envision our planet spinning on, year after year, divided into two armed groups, posed to destroy each other?

What is required to bring about changes in persistent behaviors of individuals, groups, and societies when those behaviors have become unproductive, problematic, or destructive? Or, more directly stated, What do we change; whom do we target for change; and how do we accomplish change? Should we focus our change efforts on the environment, on access to health services, on the biology of the individual, or on the individual's lifestyle? In choosing targets, shall we direct our attention toward small units—individuals—or large units—organizations or society? What strategies, or types of interventions, shall we use to accomplish change? The answer to the last question will depend both on whether our aim is first-order or second-order change and on which change strategies are appropriate in a given situation.

We will, in this section, focus on interventions that are useful in bringing about changes in persistent behaviors. We will specifically examine (1) client-intervenor relationships, (2) units of change, and (3) strategies of

Figure 4.4   *Solution to the Nine-Dot Problem*

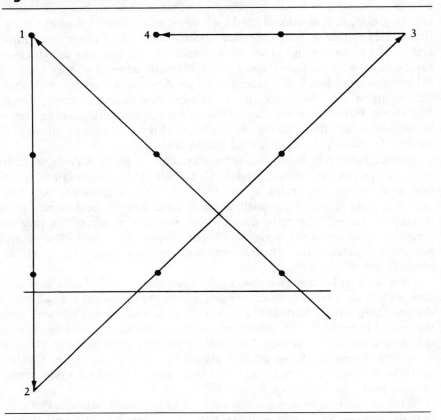

intervention. The client is the individual, group, or organization that perceives a problem and asks help in finding a solution. The intervenor (the agent of change) is the individual or group that proposes to offer a solution to the problem. The unit of change is the target population—the individual, group, or society at which efforts for change are directed. The strategy of intervention is the method of change selected by the intervenor.

Intervenors who are invited to help bring about a change in a person, a group, or an organization must first determine their opportunities for intervening to create a first- or second-order change. The model of client-intervenor relationship and the size of the unit of change will both influence that determination. The decision whether to intervene at a first- or second-order change level will direct the selection of a strategy of intervention.

The Client-Intervenor Relationship

There are three models of the client-intervenor relationship. These are the consumer, the bureaucratic, and the collaborative models.

The primary characteristic of the consumer model is that the client (the individual, group, or organization) knows what they need and seeks a purveyor of a given commodity to meet those specific needs. Thus, for an intervention to be effective, the client/consumer must be able to diagnose the problem to be changed and must be able to communicate that diagnosis to the intervenor. Further, the intervenor who is called in as a change consultant must have the skills to help facilitate the change and must be able to assess the impact of the change on the consumer. The underlying assumption of the consumer approach to intervention is the traditional view of the marketplace that "the customer is always right."

In the bureaucratic model, parties are in a client-to-professional relationship; in other words, the client surrenders responsibility for the system (individual or organizational) to the intervenor. Goodstein (1978) refers to our bureaucratic model as the medical approach, because it typifies the traditional doctor-patient relationship. He believes that the success of intervention in the bureaucratic model depends on four factors:

(a) the diagnostic skill of the consultant (recognizing that there will be little trust) and the diagnostic information made available to the consultant, which will almost always be distorted;
(b) the ability of the consultant to adequately communicate the diagnosis arrived at;
(c) the ability of the consultant to develop an adequate intervention plan based upon that diagnosis; and
(d) the ability of the consultant to carry out the intervention plan on a passive, if not resistant, client system.

The third approach, the collaborative model, is characterized by a partnership relationship between client and intervenor. The assessment of the client's needs is a shared endeavor, understood and agreed upon by both parties. The intervention is also jointly implemented by both the client and the intervenor. A commitment to collaboration by both parties is a necessary requirement, even though the intervenor may have been more involved in developing the idea for the plan, due to his or her greater familiarity with the technical aspects of implementation. Finally, the process of evaluating the outcomes of the intervention is the shared responsibility of both parties.

It should be noted that for collaboration to be successful, it must involve a commitment both to the process of participative membership and to decision making by both the intervenor and the client. Thus, collaboration is not the same as cooperation, which requires only a commitment to a shared goal and is more likely to occur in the consumer or bureaucratic models. In the collaborative model, the intervenor serves to facilitate the process of sharing and collaboration instead of focusing on a particular problem of the client system.

Units of Change

The second dimension defining interventions concerns the units of change—the systems that are the targets of efforts for change. A unit of change can be an individual, a group, an organization, a community, or a society.

Since earliest history, individuals have sought help with their problems. Groups can also be laden with many kinds of problems. Neighbors sometimes find it difficult to coexist; some work groups cannot seem to cooperate on a task; and families sometimes become estranged over the difficulties of simply living together. Organizations are large, complex groups characterized by both their task and role differentiations. They tend to be hierarchical, have expectations of how their members should behave, and require individuals to play a variety of roles. The larger and more complex the system to be changed, the more likely it is that we are confronted with an organization rather than a single group.

Larger social systems, such as communities, political units, and societies, usually contain many smaller units, such as individuals, groups, and institutions, organized into a coherent whole. We mentioned in an earlier chapter that we considered each of these units an open system, that is, a system consisting of recurrent cycles of input, transformation, and output. Although the system's input and output requirements involve dealing with the external environment, the transformation process occurs entirely within the system itself. A simple example would be a hospital with its cycle of admitting new patients and discharging those who have been successfully treated, transforming sick people into those who are on the road to recovery and discharging them into an accepting society.

We also stated earlier that all systems, or units of change, are subject to the effects of perturbations from the larger systems in which they function. This observation is true not only for the system Homo sapiens (the individual), but for all systems or units. Systems effectively resist perturbations from the outside if their transformation processes are flexible enough to adapt to these new inputs. When they are not, the system breaks down—the individual feels ill, the organization malfunctions, society is in crisis.

We believe that it is helpful to further group units of change into two categories, micro units and macro units. The value of this grouping lies in the distinction we made earlier when we referred to first-order change and second-order change. First-order change, as you will recall, refers to a change from one form of behavior to another, whereas second-order change means a change in a way of behaving. By a micro unit, we mean a unit in which change is directed to one or more components of the system with the intent that this change will result in the system's becoming more adaptable. A macro unit is a unit in which change requires the restructuring of the whole system. Later in this chapter we will explain the advantages of these categories by illustrating the uses of our developing theory of interventions. For now, however, we will present a third dimension that defines interventions: the strategy of intervention.

Strategies for Intervention

The two strategies for intervention into the affairs of others are the prescriptive approach, used in traditional public health strategies, and a second approach, based on the teaching of principles and theories to clients.

The Prescriptive Approach. Prescriptive interventions are based on the belief that the expert knows best. The intervenor provides clear directions as to how the client should go about solving the problem. The success of the intervention thus depends in large part on the intervenor's possessing sufficient knowledge and skills to allow him or her to make an accurate diagnosis and develop a plan of corrective action. Some prescriptive interventions aim at helping clients gain a better understanding of the situations in which they find themselves by providing additional information or by verifying existing data. This information is then fed back to the clients so that they can correct their misperceptions about the problem. The assumption is that the clients' problems are primarily caused by these misperceptions and that they can be corrected by the presentation of additional data.

Confrontation is a technique of the prescriptive strategy in which the intervenor presents clients with the inappropriate or invalid values by which they have been operating and then forces clients to see the unreality of these values by challenging them with facts, counter arguments, and logical explanations that encourage the clients to alter their thinking. The clients may sometimes offer their own solutions, especially if these solutions stem from a different set of values than that of the intervenor. In a special substrategy, behavior modification, the original stimulus for a client's behavioral response is linked to a new, preferable response when the intervenor presents a mode of reinforcement for the new behavior. The prescriptive approach seems to function most effectively in first-order change situations that involve changing one behavior for another.

Teaching Theory and Principles. In contrast to the prescriptive strategy, interventions based on theory and principles function on the belief that teaching clients useful theories about their behavior gives them the insight to solve both their immediate problems and other problems that may develop in the future. The advantages of teaching theories and principles is that clients learn how to understand the principles involved in solving a class of problems of which their own are only a special case. By discovering principles or rules that are outside their system and therefore useful in solving problems, clients are thus able to effect second-order change.

Central to the teaching of theory and principles is the problem of the adequacy of the instructional process. It is not easy to help people integrate their learning in such a way that they can actually use the theories in solving their own life problems. Creative and collaborative adaptations are essential in order to achieve and maintain personal and collective integrity and health in contemporary culture. The instructional process that seems most relevant to the teaching of theory and principles is the laboratory method that grew out of the cognitive field theory of learning. According to Bradford, Gibb, and Benne (1966), the founders of the laboratory movement believed that individuals were "being compelled to change by inexorable pressures from natural sciences and related technologies with little, if any preparation for handling changes, with sensitivity and effectiveness, in themselves and their relationships" (p. 35). The laboratory method of instruction was designed to fill these clients' unmet needs.

Lewin's (1948) now classic analysis of the process of planned change is the model for the laboratory approach. As you recall, he identified the first step in this process as "unfreezing." By unfreezing he meant identifying the need to give up habitual or stereotyped behaviors that are well integrated into one's behavior. All of the interventions (discussed in the previous section) that permit the client system to understand its present level of functioning and the negative consequences of this functioning can be seen as unfreezing procedures. Unfreezing also encompasses encouraging the client to consider behavioral alternatives or new norms.

Lewin's second step in planned change is "moving to a new level." New behaviors are attempted, and the client system develops some skills in these behaviors. At this point, the intervenor may need to assist the client with encouragement. Since any new set of behaviors is initially awkward and uncomfortable, the tendency to give them up and return to an older, more comfortable mode of operation is an understandable response. As we suggested earlier, the intervenor's level of activity during this phase is intensive, as he or she organizes and manages team-building workshops, skills-development programs, and other strategies to integrate the new behaviors.

The final stage of Lewin's approach to planned change is "freezing" the group's behavior at the new level. By freezing—or, actually, "refreezing" —Lewin meant the stabilization and generalization of change. In other words, the new behaviors have become part of the client's norm and are self-sustaining. In the terms of our earlier discussion, the changes that the client and the intervenor have collaboratively agreed upon have been institutionalized.

In 1946, a small group of men, principally Kurt Lewin, Leland Bradford, Kenneth Benne, and Ronald Lippitt, began to collaborate as the staff for a workshop on intergroup relations in New Britain, Connecticut. The next summer (1947) the group moved to Bethel, Maine, a place that has since become synonymous for many with the small group movement and the laboratory method of education. The founders of the first laboratory saw the group as the link between the individual and the larger social structure. The group became a medium for serving two sets of interrelated functions: (1) the reeducation of individuals toward greater integrity, better understanding of themselves and of the social conditions of their lives, including greater behavioral effectiveness in planning and achieving changes both in themselves and in their social environments, and (2) the facilitation of changes in the larger social structures upon which individual lives depend.

Can people learn to use groups for individual rehabilitation and reconstruction of the social environment? Can groups be developed that are simultaneously alive to the needs of their members for growth as persons and to the needs of the social environment for reconstruction and improvement? The founders of the laboratory answered, "Yes." The laboratory was designed as a place where people might learn, experimentally, to develop groups that would serve both purposes and, in the process, become skilled in extending similar experimental efforts into nonlaboratory settings.

Pfeiffer and Jones (1974) have provided a *Handbook of Structured Experiences for Human Relations Training,* which offers a number of structured laboratory experiences for the teacher-trainer. These experiences fall into three major categories—(1) unadapted "classic" experiences, (2) highly adapted experiences, and (3) innovative experiences—each of which serves the teacher as a model for the design of experiences that facilitate the learning of principles and theories. Blake and Moulton (1964), who offer a related approach to intervention, strongly argue that the manner in which theories are taught to the client is critical to the client's understanding and ability to put theory to future use. They further support our view that theory needs to be taught experientially if clients are to use it in their daily lives. The basic concepts of self-awareness, conflict resolution, participative decision making, and democratic leadership are examples of theory and principles best taught by the laboratory method.

Relating Interventions to First- and Second-Order Change

How would we distinguish between first- and second-order change in a real-life situation? If, for example, cigarette smokers wish to "break the habit," they may complete a program that has smoking cessation as its goal. The program may be effective in directing or convincing them to give up smoking. If it is a program based on principles of first-order change, our smokers will have replaced smoking behavior with its reciprocal, nonsmoking behavior. They will have changed from one way of behaving to another, within a given way of behaving. The given way of behaving might be a need for stress reduction or a symbol of masculinity or a symbol of feminine liberation. The symbolical meaning of these ways of behaving will, of course, differ from smoker to smoker depending on his or her life history.

These ways of behaving can also be seen as representing personal values. *Value* is a good descriptive term to use, since values are usually defined as guides to a large number of individual behaviors. Because these ways of behaving are based on individual values, they reflect personal lifestyles. Our smokers have changed one behavior for another but have not changed their personal value systems. The program has indeed helped our smokers to accomplish their goal, namely, to stop smoking. Many people involved in this type of first-order-change program find this outcome quite acceptable. It should be made clear, however, that first-order change will not actually solve the problem: our smokers may find that six months later they are again smoking. Or, they may cease smoking and replace this habit with gulping down several doughnuts and several cups of coffee a day, resulting in jittery nerves and a large weight gain. Their doctors may note the change by documenting that they have gone down in one risk factor, smoking, only to go up in others, including obesity.

In contrast, second-order change would aim at helping smokers to change their lifestyles rather than substituting one behavior for another. That is, a program based on second-order-change principles would promote change in those personal values that guide or inform the lifestyle of the smoker. Consequently, the program planners would need to recognize that the smoking behavior is a manifestation of a certain kind of lifestyle rather than a specific behavior (smoking) that needs to be changed. It is possible that the failure of many programs aimed at smoking cessation are due to this misperception on the part of the program planners.

An Evolving Theory of Change

We are now ready to put together the pieces of our "change puzzle" and observe how our theory of change looks. The various pieces of our puzzle include, first, the concepts of first- and second-order change (their practical application in terms of change from one behavior to another behavior, as opposed to change from one way of behaving to another) and, second, the three dimensions of intervention: the client-intervenor relationship, the units of change, and the strategies of intervention.

Table 4.1   *Types and Levels of Change*

	Micro Change	Macro Change	Change Strategies
First-order change	Individual change from one behavior to another	Organizational change from one behavior to another	Prescriptive: 1. Informational 2. Confrontive 3. Directive
Second-order change	Individual change in ways of behaving	Community/ society change in ways of behaving	Teaching theory and principles by laboratory method.

For the sake of clarity, we have outlined this change puzzle in Table 4.1. The units of change (micro and macro) and types of change strategies are at the top of the table, and the two levels of change (first- and second-order) are on the sides of the table. Reading the table across, you will observe that first-order change is applicable to both individuals and organizations (i.e., to both micro and macro units). Each of the three prescriptive strategies can be seen as an applicable intervention to accomplish first-order change with either kind of unit. The bottom part of the table shows that second-order change can be used with both individuals and the large social units of community and society. The change strategy of choice used to achieve second-order change is the teaching of theories and principles.

Change Theory in Practice: A Case Illustration

Having summarized our evolving theory of change, we will now examine the application of change theory to actual practice. The case we have selected will address the four questions that evolve from our theory of change: (1) what to change, (2) whom to change, (3) the choice of type of change, and (4) how to create the change. We can answer the first with the change formula presented in Chapter 1,

$$Hs = (f)\ E + AcHS + B + Ls$$

which state that health status is a function of the environment, access to health services, biological factors, and lifestyle. In other words, in order to change health status, we must change the elements in the formula. The second issue, who to change, concerns our choice of change targets, specifically, the individual, the organization, or the society. The third issue, the type of change, is concerned with the choice of either a first- or second-order change. Finally, the fourth issue raises the question of which change strategy is appropriate—the prescriptive approach or the teaching of theory and principles.

Introduction to the Case.   In recent years occupational health issues have received increasing attention, primarily because of recent findings related to chemical carcinogenicity and hazardous exposures in the workplace. The tasks of occupational health specialists, educators, and investigators are to identify the diseases and conditions that result from exposures or conditions in the workplace, to recommend changes to eliminate these conditions, and to assign responsibility for effecting these changes.

In our case, health educators have been asked to develop some options for improving the health status of a group of women who are employed as sewers and stitchers in garment factories in Worcester, Massachusetts. After reviewing what is known about the musculoskeletal disorder *carpal tunnel syndrome* (CTS) and examining a project currently underway in the International Ladies' Garment Workers Union (ILGWU) in Worcester, Massachusetts, we will examine possible change strategies within the garment industry and their impact on both employers and employees.

Overview of the Problem.   Carpal tunnel syndrome (CTS) results from pressure on the median nerve, which passes through the space between the carpal, or wrist, bones. When this nerve is compressed within the space between the wrist bones as the result of irritation or an inflammation, movement is inhibited in the thumb and first two fingers of the hand. The common symptoms of CTS are nighttime tingling and numbness of the thumb and first two fingers, clumsiness of the affected hand, and muscular wasting of the thumb. CTS is a progressive disorder, which, if left untreated, may result in complete hand disability.

In medical literature, CTS has been associated with certain systemic diseases, such as diabetes, acromegaly, and rheumatoid arthritis. The syndrome occurs most commonly in middle-aged women. Certain occupational factors have also been associated with CTS, including repetitive hand motion and low-frequency vibrations.

Currently, musculoskeletal disorders found in the women of Worcester Local 75 of the ILGWU are being studied by health personnel at the University of Massachusetts Medical Center, which has recently contracted to perform physical exams for union members as part of their health benefits package, and by faculty of the Harvard School of Public Health. The ILGWU is of particular interest in the study of CTS because most of its members are high-risk, middle-aged women whose jobs require repetitive hand motions. The design of the Worcester study is cross-sectional, and information is being collected on physical symptoms, employment history, and personal factors by means of a self-administered questionnaire. Individuals who indicate the presence of hand symptoms will be evaluated for physical signs of CTS.

Although the ILGWU shops in Worcester vary in size, degree of modernization, and types of garment manufactured, the predominant job task in all shops is machine operation, or stitching. In the future, all job tasks will be analyzed by a team of experienced biomechanists, but even to an untrained eye, the job of stitching appears to require wrist flexion, repetitive motion, and forceful manipulation of the fabric. It is too early to speculate on the results of this study, but let's assume that repetitive motion is causally related to CTS and that CTS can be proven to be an occupational disease. Given these assumptions, the important question is, How can the occurrence of CTS among garment workers be decreased?

Evaluating Options for Change. If the results were to show a significantly higher rate of CTS among machine operators than among other workers, possible options would be (1) to change the way the stitchers and sewers work, so that stress on the wrist is reduced, or (2) to change the physical arrangement of the sewing machine and work table. Let's evaluate these options using our model of change.

Training individuals to work in such a way that they will exert less stress on their wrists is an example of first-order micro change (i.e., substituting one behavior for another). Each new employee could be trained in these new work methods, and health educators could arrange seminars and workshops to illustrate the types of hand motions that contribute to CTS. The employer would benefit since fewer workers would be absent because of hand and wrist pain, and might even gain long-term benefits if fewer workers develop compensable cases of CTS. The problem with this type of change is that switching one form of behavior to another may, in fact, give rise to new disorders if, for example, movements and pressures are transferred from the wrist to the elbow and shoulder. Another problem is that the change puts responsibility for the condition on the workers, along with implicit blame: "... if you worked correctly, this wouldn't have happened in the first place."

Second-order micro change, or lifestyle change, would involve changing worker attitudes toward their work. The idea is that if the women recognize that their work as machine operators puts them at risk of developing CTS, they will change from passive acceptance of the current mode of production to a more self-assertive and self-reliant attitude. This change in attitude would enhance their freedom of choice. They may, for example, ask for retraining and assignment to a different job, or they may decide that the time is right to organize collectively and negotiate with their employer to change their work conditions (thus instituting a macro change).

Redesigning the sewing machine and work table according to ergonomic theory would be a viable option for change if biomechanic specialists determined that these factors were contributing to repetitive trauma. This action would be an example of first-order macro change. The employer, having been told that the design of the workspace is faulty, would initiate organizational changes that would alter the structural layout of the shop. Such a use of an outside expert to redesign the workplace illustrates a prescriptive strategy. The employers would modify the shop because they have gained new information suggesting that the changes are needed to help alleviate the problem of CTS.

The two change strategies we've just discussed would be adequate if the occurrence of CTS can be shown to be related causally to individual methods of working or to the physical design of the workplace, in a linear one-to-one relationship. It is more likely, however, that CTS is a result of several occupational and personal factors and that simply substituting one behavior for another, whether on the part of employer or employee, will not eliminate the problem. The roots of the problem most likely have their origin in the interaction of employer, employees, and the workplace. One manifestation of this interaction, for example, is the salary schedule of the union employees, in which workers are paid according to the piecework method. Wages per shift are calculated according to the number of garments produced. Such a system of compensation encourages workers to work as quickly and efficiently as possible. Thus, as workers adopt styles of working that allow them to bring home their desired pay, it is not inconceivable that some workers have adopted methods involving repetitive wrist motions that place them at high risk of developing CTS. Training these workers in a less hazardous work method might have some impact on occurrence of CTS, but if the true incentive of higher wages remains, these training sessions may have little impact on the problem. Similarly, redesigning the workspace may help relieve the pressure on the wrist but could easily turn out to be an empty gesture on the part of the employer if the pay system is not also changed.

What requires changing in this instance is the piecework salary. This action would be an example of second-order macro change. To create such a change, both employer and employee would have to understand the theory and principles underlying the need to change to another mode of compensation, as well as the reasons for certain workers' maladaptations in work methods. Although it might appear at the outset that both parties would lose money and that nothing would be gained immediately, the long-term outcome would benefit both—fewer cases of CTS in the workplace, fewer days lost from work, and treatment of the underlying problem causing CTS rather than its symptoms. Table 4.2 summarizes the change options and strategies we have just discussed.*

---

*We owe much of this case presentation to Adele Miller, who collected the data and prepared the analysis in Table 4.2.

Table 4.2 Options for Change to Reduce Carpel Tunnel Syndrome

	First-Order Change	Strategy	Second-Order Change	Strategy
Micro Change	Change worker behavior to reduce wrist strain.	Supply information to worker; worker practices new movements	Workers change ways of behaving to 1. Ask for reassignment to new job; 2. Organize collectively to negotiate to change work conditions.	Teach theory and principles of participative membership and participative decision making.
Macro Change	Change organizational behavior by redesigning machine and work table.	Outside expert prescribes machine redesign.	Industry changes ways of behaving to 1. Eliminate piecework as a competitive incentive system; 2. Develop collaboration to act as an incentive system.	Teach theory and principles, including "Z" theory of management,* on industry-wide basis.

Note: *The "Z" theory of management concerns the development of collaborative management approaches to problems of plant management.

The Effect of Social Values on Choice of Level of Change

In Chapter 3, we were concerned with the problem of what needs to be changed to ensure improved health status among members of a society. In that chapter we stated that the social values held by members of a society both define the forms that the health care delivery system assumes and establishes the boundaries and directions along which the system may be acceptably modified. We further referred to four social values basic to the health care system: personal responsibility, social concern, freedom, and equality. We also categorized the two major attitudes that people hold concerning each of these values as libertarian and egalitarian. Libertarians emphasize personal achievement and the freedom of the individual; egalitarians are primarily concerned with equality of opportunity, and perceive freedom as a means for equalizing these opportunities for choice.

We are now ready to explain how social values affect the choice of the direction and level of change that will be pursued by change agents in the health care system. The change options we discussed with regard to the problem of CTS among workers in the garment industry demonstrate that a variety of choices is potentially possible. Our position is that the choices of "who will be changed" and the "order of change" are largely based on the social values of the relevant decision makers. For example, as Figure 4.5 demonstrates, we believe that first-order change is consistent with libertarian social values. The arrows in the figure represent the general direction of social change perceived as desirable by those individuals holding libertarian social values. The downward direction signifies reducing the pressure on organizations and social systems for change, while putting the responsibility to change on individuals. The horizontal arrow denotes reducing all second-order change directed at individuals, therefore reducing the likelihood that changes in attitudes and values in individuals may lead to major changes in organizations and social systems.

Figure 4.5 *The Effect of Libertarian Values on Choice of Options for Change*

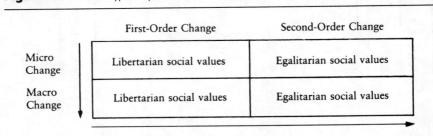

	First-Order Change	Second-Order Change
Micro Change	Libertarian social values	Egalitarian social values
Macro Change	Libertarian social values	Egalitarian social values

Egalitarians prefer to encourage both organizations and society to take
more social responsibility. If increased social responsibility is to be translated into action, then members of society must emphasize the need for
second-order change in organizations and society. In Figure 4.6, for example, the direction of the arrows represents the egalitarian view of social
change: less emphasis on individual responsibility to change (the upward
arrow) and greater emphasis on the responsibility of organizations and
society to initiate and support change (the horizontal arrow). Developing
second-order change options would increase the possibilities for changes
in lifestyle and for major organizational and societal changes.

To illustrate the effect of social values on the choice of the order of
change and on those change strategies employed by the health educator
practitioner, we can return to our example of how to reduce the risk of
CTS faced by workers in the garment industry. In Table 4.2 we reviewed
four options for change upon which health educators could base a program of risk reduction for this population. We suggest that the relevant
decision makers, in this case the employer, the union, and the health
educators, will make their decision based on several factors (the costs and
benefits of each option, the availability of resources, and so on), and that
one of the often overlooked but most important factors will be the social
values of the decision makers—their underlying beliefs about freedom,
equality, social concern, and personal responsibility.

Looking at Table 4.3 (p. 86), let's examine more closely the four possible strategies for change and the social values that inform the choice of
each option. The table makes clear that first-order changes are based on a
libertarian view of social values, whereas egalitarian attitudes underlie
both second-order micro and macro change. For example, in Table 4.3 we
refer to a first-order macro change in which the employer is instructed to
redesign the sewing machine and work table to alleviate behaviors leading

Figure 4.6   *The Effect of Egalitarian Values on Choice of Options for Change*

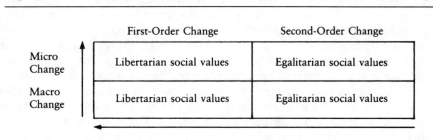

	First-Order Change	Second-Order Change
Micro Change	Libertarian social values	Egalitarian social values
Macro Change	Libertarian social values	Egalitarian social values

Table 4.3 *Social Values Underlying Options for Change to Reduce Carpel Tunnel Syndrome*

	First-Order Change	Second-Order Change
Micro Change	**Action:** Instruct workers how to use hand motions that will not result in CTS.	**Action:** Facilitate the development of self-reliance and initiative in workers so that they are able to work toward macro change or retrain for new jobs
	Social value (Libertarian): Workers are responsible for their own health; they should change their hand motions or suffer the consequence of disability.	**Social value (Egalitarian):** Once workers have developed an attitude of self-reliance, they have the freedom to make alternative choices, i.e., retrain for a new job or organize for a change in conditions.
Macro Change	**Action:** The employer is instructed to redesign the sewing machine and work table to alleviate motions leading to CTS.	**Action:** Organize workers and employers to work together to eliminate piecework pay and to replace it with an adequate salary.
	Social value (Libertarian): The employer has the responsibility to modify the shop and alleviate the work situation leading to CTS and thereby increase worker productivity.	**Social value (Egalitarian):** The legal guarantee of the right to collective action to achieve change is based on the notion of the government as an expression of the public will.

to CTS. In employing this change option the employer assumes the responsibility to modify the shop so that worker behavior will be less likely to lead to CTS, thereby both reducing his employer compensation costs and increasing worker productivity. This change option is consonant with the libertarian social value of personal responsibility. An example of a change option supported by holders of egalitarian social values would be second-order macro change. The change action in this case would involve organizing workers to negotiate with the employer to eliminate piecework pay and to replace it with an adequate salary. The egalitarian social value held by the workers who have in this case decided to organize is the legal guarantee of the right to collectively achieve change. This is a right that the government grants to the people as an expression of the public will.

In the United States support for changes in the health care system in the twentieth century has come mainly from governmental bodies. The two major parties, the Democrats and the Republicans, have traditionally represented opposing sets of social values: the Democrats are usually considered to foster egalitarian views; the Republicans, a libertarian perspective. For example, the egalitarian social values of the Carter administration led their spokespersons in health care to endorse health promotion and prevention as goals of health care. These Carter appointees defined health promotion as reducing the risk to the individual through developing individual responsibility to manage smoking behavior, alcohol and drug consumption, and stress, and to increase personal fitness. Their strategies for health prevention included educating individuals to take personal responsibility for family planning, pregnancy, and infant care, and for reduction in risk behaviors leading to stroke and coronary heart disease. These goals call for second-order micro changes. (However, even in the administration's definitive statement of goals for change, *Healthy People,* [1979] the Surgeon General did not endorse second-order macro change.) In contrast, the Republican Reagan administration, committed to a libertarian perspective, has considerably reduced federal moneys and support for second-order changes. Instead their spokespersons on health care have affirmed the freedom of individuals to choose to live in either healthy or unhealthy conditions and to seek support for either first- or second-order micro change, if such support is available in the private sector.

Ethical Dilemmas in Behavior Change

In the preceding sections, we have outlined a theory of change that we consider important to the effective practice of health education. Trying to implement changes, however, raises significant ethical issues for the agent of change. We will now review some of these issues, look at the ethical dilemmas they pose, and discuss their implications for practitioners of behavior change.

For several reasons, contemporary educators, particularly those involved in the practice and investigation of behavior change, are becoming increasingly more aware of the ethical dilemmas posed by their activities. First, our knowledge about the control of human behavior is rapidly increasing. Second, there is a readiness within our society to use methods that work, without much concern for either long-term consequences or short-run effects of these efforts. Third, both educators and social scientists concerned with behavior change are becoming increasingly useful to

many agencies within government, industry, and fields of public health
and social welfare. It has been suggested that possibilities now exist
for our new knowledge to be used to control and manipulate human
behavior.

This potential power to control human behavior creates a dilemma for
the practitioner and investigator of behavior change. For example, those
who hold to the basic democratic value of freedom of choice must inevitably see any manipulation of the behavior of others as a violation of human rights. This would be their position regardless of the "goodness" of
the cause or the form of the manipulation. On the other hand, there are
many situations in which most of us would consider behavior change a
desirable goal, particularly if the result is the maintenance of wellness or
the improvement of health status. We see educational interventions as particularly beneficial in achieving these goals—but can those interventions
be accomplished without some form of behavior manipulation or control?
This question illustrates the two horns of the dilemma. Although the
manipulation of behavior may violate one of our fundamental values,
there is no way to structure an effective change situation so that manipulation does not occur, at least to some degree.

Given this quandry, how should health educators engage in health-related behavioral change? The field of health education is a relative new-
comer to the health professions, and it is only in recent years that health
educators have become increasingly concerned about ethics and the need
for ethical standards. We may consider Kleinschmidt and Zimand's (1953)
statement as a benchmark "in establishing ethical awareness within this
profession." "It is very important," they stressed, "that the health educator consider seriously what he is doing to the minds of people when he
undertakes to influence them" (p. 23).

Health educators have been especially concerned with the change
strategies employed in the pursuit of their professional goals. The typolo-
gy of change strategies we have developed views social intervention on a
continuum, with coercion represented by decisions handed down by outside experts at one extreme and facilitation through the teaching of theory
and principles at the other. The methods of persuasion and dissemination
of information are represented as points in between these extremes. The
central question is, Do some or all of these strategies violate the rights of
those targeted for change?

One possible solution to this question is to apply change strategies only
if the targeted individual or group has volunteered to participate in the
program. But does "voluntary" always mean "free choice"? Ruth and Al-
lan Faden (1978) have suggested that the degree of "voluntariness" with
which a client responds can depend on the amount of relevant information the client possesses about both the health issue under concern and the
possible alternatives.

A second, related solution to the issue of individual rights centers around the notion of informed consent. For example, in principle two of its Code of Ethics, the Society for Public Education states that "health educators observe the principle of informed consent with respect to individuals and groups served." Many health educators believe that "informed consent" is a way out of the dilemma between freedom of choice and manipulation. They assert that the consumer has a free choice only after he or she has been given all the information necessary to make such a choice. We question this belief for several reasons. First, the Faden's criticisms of voluntariness point to the difficulty of pinning down the concepts of voluntary and involuntary participation. Second, there is evidence that many health educators do not generally trust the idea of informed consent; if they did, wouldn't they also be forced to believe in "informed nonconsent"? Informed nonconsent implies that the consumer, once fully informed, may have reason to choose to refuse to follow a specific health behavior. How many health professionals, however, give as much information against as well as in support of nonsmoking, Pap smears, family planning, or any other health-related action they are trying to promote? If we are honest, we must admit that most of us are more informative and more persuasive in presenting the behaviors in which we believe.

Are we, then, to remain forever caught in the dilemma? Or are there some ethical guidelines that can help us move forward? Although Kelman (1969), in an essay on value dilemmas and behavior change, believes that no real resolution of the dilemma is possible, he does offer some ways of mitigating the effects of manipulation. He suggests three steps:

(1) Increasing our own and others' active awareness of the manipulative aspects of our work and the ethical ambiquities inherent therein;
(2) deliberately building protection against manipulation or resistance to it into the processes we use or study; and
(3) setting the enhancement of freedom of choices as a central positive goal for our practice and research (p. 591).

When we translate Kelman's three steps into practice, we find that providing health information need not present a major ethical problem if we clearly follow the guidance suggested in step one. Specifically, we need to be aware of our particular biases as they are reflected in the manner of our presentation and in the possible omission of significant facts. In addition, persuasion does not offer serious difficulties as long as the targets of persuasion willingly listen to us. The key word is "willingly." Kelman's steps two and three can serve as significant reminders of our ethical responsibilities when we consider using methods that are designed to weaken an individual's ability to resist manipulation and control.

From this point of view, the use of behavior modification is a particularly sensitive issue. This method has come into wide use in client education. It may well be ethically justifiable if clients knowingly expose themselves to behavioral modification techniques with the expectation that these techniques will help them do what they want. However, when behavior modification is used without or against a person's will, it becomes a violation of his or her rights.

Should we, in the interest of the health goals of the profession, proselytize for these goals without honoring a person's right to resist? At least two issues are involved in this question. First, health educators have, in fact, urged people to follow recommended health practices that were later rescinded. At one time, for example, health educators persuaded people to have chest X-rays at mobile units every six months. Only later did they learn that this practice needlessly exposed the public to the even greater danger of radiation. The second issue is that, even if we are certain about the benefits of a given health measure, people still retain the right to resist our efforts. For example, we recognize that a number of health-related behaviors, among them habits concerning smoking, exercise, eating, and the use of alcohol, still remain in the domain of an individual's free choice.

But if we *strictly* adhered to Kelman's emphasis on freedom of choice, would we not possibly swing too far in the direction of the endorsement of individual rights? Certainly, society as a whole has justifiable concerns. The unlimited freedom of any one person may well abridge other person's freedom. It is generally accepted that if we wish to preserve everyone's rights, then all people must accept certain restrictions on their own behavior. We also accept the idea that no individual or group should be allowed to engage in actions that pose serious threats to the health, safety, and welfare of others (for example, contaminate the water or pollute the air we breathe). It is clear that the health professions have the responsibility to identify such behaviors and work toward changing them through education and regulation.

Perhaps the best general rule to follow for interpreting Kelman's three steps is to give priority to the individual's right to adopt or not adopt a recommended behavior where the problem affects only the individual and not the health of others. When, however, individual or organizational behaviors threaten the health and welfare of others, health educators have the choice of using education, or possibly regulation, to stop this behavior.

The profession of health education is just beginning to move toward developing guidelines of ethical behavior that relate to the dilemmas we have been discussing and to the questions of professional preparation and professional accountability. In 1976 the Society for Public Health Education adopted a code of ethics; and in 1979 the Association for the Advancement of Health Education sponsored a Conference on Ethical Issues in Health Education, which identified ethical issues in the areas of professional preparation, methods, research, accountability, and political activities. The code of ethics adopted in 1976 set standards that were agreed upon by some but not all health educators. These standards are reflected in the following nine principles from the code:

1. Health educators do not discriminate because of race, color, religion, age, sex, national ancestry or socioeconomic status in rendering service, hiring, promotion, or training.
2. Health educators observe the principle of informed consent with respect to individuals and groups served.
3. Health educators value privacy, dignity, and the worth of the individual, and use skills consistent with these values.
4. Health educators maintain their competence at the highest levels through continuing study, training, and research.
5. Health educators foster an educational environment which nurtures individual growth and development.
6. Health educators support change by choice, not by coercion.
7. Health educators as researchers or practitioners report activities and findings honestly and without distortion.
8. Health educators accurately represent their competence, education, training, and experience and act within the boundaries of their professional competence.
9. Health educators are aware of unprofessional practices, and are accountable for taking appropriate action to eliminate these practices.

In conclusion, we concur with the summary statement of Barnes *et al.* (1980) in their article on ethical issues: "Perhaps to some, the unwieldy process of debating philosophy and ethics and attempting to arrive at a consensus may seem wasteful and unproductive. However, if there is a heightened awareness of the need for caution and care in regulating our conduct, we will have evolved, as a profession, to a higher level of wellness" (p. 9).

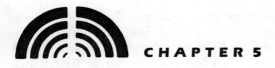

CHAPTER 5

Understanding Health Education Practice

Where does health education take place? If we wanted to see a health educator in practice, where would we look? Does health education occur only in schools and doctors' offices? What are the characteristics of those settings in which it does occur? Are there any relationships between types of settings and the kinds of health education that take place in those settings?

A logical way to begin to answer these questions is to develop an operational definition of health education. In Chapter 2 we developed an evolving definition of health education as a process involving change in the health-related behaviors and lifestyles of individuals and groups. However, because health education is more than a process, we are now prepared to add an "operational dimension" to our definition; that is, to expand our definition to include all important determinants of health education practice and the ways in which these variables come together to bring about a health education outcome. Once we have done this, we will develop a model for health education practice in order to explain the distribution of health education programs within a given setting and to define those skills necessary for practice.

Toward an Operational Definition of Health Education

The Problem of Defining Health Education

Two factors about health education have, at times, been troublesome for the health education profession. These are, first, that health education can occur anywhere and, second, that nearly everyone believes they can do it. Because of these factors, the development of an operational definition of health education has remained elusive. If health education is difficult to define and can occur anywhere, and if virtually anyone can do it, people ask, Why do we need health education programs or, for that matter, health education specialists? (Health education specialists are defined as those persons with specialized skills and competencies in health education practice. Chapter 9 will discuss these ideas in detail, as well as the notion that health education is indeed a profession.)

Our problem can be further traced to two more difficulties. First, process definitions of health education do not specify how to change health-related behaviors, nor do they state what skills are necessary to become effective health educators. Second, because we live in a product-oriented, technocratic society, we tend to quantify almost everything. We go to school to "get an education." We work to "get paid" so we can "buy food and housing." When we are sick, we visit a clinic or hospital to "get well." We live in a society that not only reinforces a quantitative perspective on life but leaves us with few choices other than to obtain necessary goods and services in the marketplace. To ensure good measure, we take great pains to count and quantify each unit we receive.

Given the quantitative climate in which health educators must function, it is easy to see why they, as a group, have had difficulty explaining the meaning of health (in contrast to the meaning of medical care) and have struggled to explain what it means to be a "health-educated person." In a sense, health educators have remained idealists in a pragmatic world. They have resisted quantification of their activities and have continued to maintain that "health education cannot be given to one person by another," and that "it is not a set of procedures to be carried out or a product to be achieved"' Rather, "it is a dynamic, ever changing process of development in which a person is accepting or rejecting new information, new attitudes, new practices concerned with the objectives of healthful living" (Bureau of Health Education, 1980, p. 1).

To be an effective practitioner, it is important to recognize that any definition of health education must include not only the process but also the understanding that health education functions in direct relationship with the setting in which it occurs and the external environment in which it exists.

How Does a Person Become Health Educated?

What does it mean to speak of health education occurring in a setting and to say that the setting is itself part of a larger environment? To answer this question it is first necessary to understand how an individual enters a setting that offers health education services. Most individuals are more familiar with entry into a setting that offers education rather than entry into a medical care setting; in fact, both processes involve a complex set of behaviors exhibited over a period of time on the part of the consumers of health care. First, they must determine that they need "medical care" or "an education." Second, they must transform this desire into action by evaluating the alternative places or settings that provide these services. Third, they must initiate contact with a specific institution that will provide those services. Fourth, at an appointed time, they must arrive at the setting and move through an elaborate maze of procedures to attain their goals.

In a medical care setting, these procedures might involve answering questions for a medical history, having a physical examination, or having a blood test or an X-ray taken. Such activities may occur only once, or many times. In contrast, an educational setting might require a person to visit three times a week for anywhere from four to nine months up to four to six years, with a possible series of interrelated coursework. "Becoming educated" may involve reading books, learning another language, writing papers or exams, or solving elaborate math problems with a computer. In both instances, however, the person ultimately ends up with a list of procedures that must be followed. Briefly, in the medical setting such procedures are called *prescriptions* (a list of activities a person should do to improve his or her health). In an educational setting, these procedures are referred to as a *curriculum* (a list of all courses necessary to graduate).

The essential point is that when we say we want to "get well" or "become educated," we are usually describing the process of interacting with an elaborate institution or system. These interactions with institutions of medical care or education are the goods and services we desire. In this "marketplace" we exchange money for the services of the institution. The transaction is recorded in the elaborate social accounting system that society has developed to measure who receives what or does what to whom.

Process Versus Outcome

The outcome we seek from our interaction with health or educational institutions is not goods or services but rather to become healthy or to become educated. However, the fact remains that we cannot obtain wellness or get an education from any external source. In other words, we must recognize that all individuals have the power to accept or reject their own education or their own healing. Both outcomes are ultimately the result of do-it-yourself propositions. In simple terms, doctors "doctor," but it is the body itself that heals. Dr. William H. Hazlett has said that he believes "there is a quality in people yet untapped that can be awakened and allowed to flower, but neither the politicians nor the medical people have found it, probably because the former looks upon health as a commodity, the latter as service to be rendered, and neither as something a person may aspire to and realize." The quality Hazlett refers to is an understanding of the relationship between the mind and the body.

Of course, if we are sick, taking medicine or following a physician's advice can often assist the body to heal more quickly. If we are not diseased, that is, if we are not suffering from a maladaptation of our body in its attempt to counter stimuli or stresses that impinge on us, however, there is very little a physician can do to make us "more healthy." In a similar manner, teachers "teach," but it is an active, involved mind that enables one to learn. In fact, in many cases a student will learn more outside a classroom, reading in the library or talking with friends, than from only attending classes three times a week.

The idea that the activities of becoming healthy or becoming educated focus on internal mind-body relationships means that both can occur either with or without a specific interaction with a medical or educational institution. Each may happen anywhere, and anyone may be able to help us "do them" (to assist our bodies to heal, or our minds to learn). However, because our society places value on both educated and healthy people, we have organized social institutions designed to assist people in pursuing their goals of becoming healthy and educated. Some of us use these institutions because we are taught by our heritage to value them. Others of us decide for ourselves that they are convenient to, or valuable for, our purposes. The important function of these institutions, whether hospitals, colleges, or their less traditional counterparts, is that they serve as facilitators of the internal mind-body processes that lead us to the outcomes we desire.

Health Education Operationally Defined

When we say that most definitions of health education are process definitions, we mean that they attempt to describe the nature of the mind-body internalization that occurs as a person grows or learns but that they fail to include the concepts of "structure" or "outcome" as necessary components of health education. By adding these components, we can evolve from a process definition to one with "operational" dimensions. Our operational definition is that health education is (1) a planned opportunity to learn about health, (2) which occurs in a setting, (3) at a given point in time, and (4) involves an interaction between teacher(s) and learner(s).

"Learning about health" may occur either spontaneously, as a function of a particular interaction between two or more persons, or as a deliberate, planned activity (called a program) on the part of either the health professional, the consumer, or both. The idea that learning about health can occur during a deliberate, planned intervention distinguishes the field of health education from other health disciplines. Thus, it is important to understand that a planned educational intervention (a health education program), in contrast to a spontaneous learning event, has known objectives and methods that are believed to produce specific behavioral outcomes. The design of these educational interventions forms the basis for health education practice within any setting.

Health educators recognize that individual learning does not occur in a random pattern. In fact, learning follows specific, characteristic patterns that can be both understood and measured. Human curiosity is the fundamental motivation of health education, as it is in any scientific discipline. Health educators' curiosity is focused on why and how people learn about health and illness. They wonder how some people learn to take preventive actions when others do not. How do certain people learn to assume responsibility for their health while others do not? When, where, how, and why does learning about health occur? Health educators seek answers to these questions in order to develop educational interventions that will prevent disease or alter the impact of disease.

Health Education Programs as Planned Educational Interventions

Health educators recognize that as individuals interact with their environment, they are exposed to many opportunities for learning about how to "become healthy." Most of these learning opportunities occur spontaneously in conversations with family or friends in their homes. Others occur at work or school as individuals pursue their daily activities. Although nearly all settings provide some potential for learning opportunities related to health, health educators believe that some settings provide greater potential than others. For example, when people are visiting a physician's office because they are ill, their attention is very likely to be focused on a specific complaint or problem. They are motivated, at some level, to learn, because they have voluntarily sought assistance of medical providers in solving their problem (i.e., to become healthy again). During the time immediately before and after their visit, these people are likely to be very receptive to information about their specific problem and to those actions they might take to prevent the problem from recurring.

The Concept of a Learning Opportunity: Theory and Practice

Timeliness and setting, however, are not the only important variables that affect whether or not learning about health will occur. The potential for a learning opportunity in a given setting also depends on the person who does the teaching and that person's effectiveness in communicating with the learner. In addition, the learners themselves bring to the "teaching moment" not only the specific problem but also many other internal and external influences on their lives, as well as all their previous experi-

Table 5.1 *A Formula for Expressing the Potential of a Given
Learning Opportunity*

$$LO_p = (f)\ S + T + Ed\ (N{:}O{:}M{:}E) + Ln$$

where

LO_p = the *potential* for a *learning opportunity* during which a
person is receptive to learning in a given setting.

(f) = some *function* or combination of the following independent
variables.

S = a given *setting* where the learning might occur.

T = the appropriateness, or *timeliness,* of the moment.

Ed = the educator or teacher.

$(N{:}O{:}M{:}E)$ = the abililty of the educator to define the *needs* of the
learner, establish behavioral *objectives,* provide appropriate
methods, and *evaluate* the learning that occurred.

Ln = the *learner* or student.

ences with the setting. We have restated these variables associated with
the given potential of a learning opportunity in the formula in Table 5.1.

What, then, is the probability of a given individual learning about
health? At this point it might be helpful to provide an example of how the
concept of the "potential of a given learning opportunity" may be applied
in a practical manner. Consider this description of an appropriately designed and executed health education program, which occurred in eastern
Kentucky.

When the clinic first opened, many of the mountain people, who for
years, had stoically endured illness and pain simply because they had
no alternative, rushed to the clinic's emergency room on the slightest
pretext. But Stumbo (the clinic physician) and his coworkers could not
afford to cater to the whims of patients who wanted to sit back pas-
sively and let the doctor take care of their problems. They immediately
began the process of educating the patients. "Once a mother had come
into the emergency room, we had her," Jan Stumbo recalls. "We could
educate her. If she brought in a feverish child in the middle of the
night, we would hand her a thermometer and teach her how to use it,
explain to her what a fever was and teach her when to call the doctor
right away and when to wait until morning." The number of emergency calls has dropped from 15 or 20 a week when the clinic first opened
to about one a night (Hening, 1976, pp. 24–27).

Here, the specific problem was overuse or inappropriate use of medical
services in an emergency room. The problem resulted in higher costs to
the facility (provision of staff and equipment) and to patients (higher costs

per visit, great concern for illness). The problem was resolved through a planned educational intervention.

We can apply our formula for a learning opportunity from Table 5.1 to examine this program. The setting (S) was the emergency room; the time (T) was during an emergency visit; the educator (Ed) was a nurse; and the learner (Ln) was the mother of a sick child. The planned educational intervention involved (N) a need (the mother's lack of knowledge and skills to determine her child's degree of illness); (O) an objective (to change the behavior of mothers regarding their sick children and teach appropriate use of physician and emergency room services); (M) a method (instruction by the nurse, along with the gift of a thermometer); and (E) an evaluation (done by determining an outcome of "appropriate use" and using trend analysis to document whether change actually occurred. We'll look further at this type of measurement, a simple before-and-after evaluation design, in Chapter 8.

In our Kentucky example, the potential for a given learning opportunity was high. It was apparent that the learner, with her sick child, had an obvious concern. Her belief that her child was ill served as a motivating factor in her readiness to learn and adopt a new behavior. Thus, the timeliness of the intervention was very appropriate: if the intervention had occurred at a time when the child was well, the mother might have had less concern. The setting also served to reinforce this opportunity, by allowing the educator (the nurse) to be available because of a flexible schedule that gave her time to teach the patient. Finally, the program or educational intervention was specific to a given problem and target population, had clearly stated objectives, made use of methods that were sensitive to the culture (e.g., provision of a thermometer when most mothers could not afford to buy them), and was evaluated using measurable outcomes. Had any of these variables been different, the potential for the learning opportunity would also have been different. For example, an important ingredient of the successful outcome was the recognized need for adequately trained nursing staff present in the emergency room. This factor assured that the program could occur. Had the nurses not been available, treatment without education would have been the outcome. The problem of emergency room misuse would no doubt have continued.

Predicting a Health Education Outcome

Now that we have developed a conceptual model of a learning opportunity that can occur in a given setting, we can use this model to answer the questions posed at the end of the last section. Why is it that certain people learn to assume responsibility for their health while others do not? A health educator might rephrase this question by asking, What is the likelihood that a planned, deliberately, structured, educational intervention will change an individual's behavior or lifestyle? Written as a formula, the answer to this question appears in Table 5.2.

Table 5.2 *A Formula for Expressing the Probability of a Given Health Education Outcome*

$$Ln_{heo} = (f)\, LO_n + LO_{eff}$$

where

Ln_{heo} = the dependent variable *health education outcome* (e.g., behavioral change, lifestyle change, institutional change or societial change). It is the probability that a given person or learner (*Ln*) (or target of change) will, in fact, change.

LO_n = the *number* of deliberately structured *learning opportunities* to which the learner is exposed, in a given setting, or the sum of learning opportunities that have occurred in two or more settings.

LO_{eff} = the rated *effectiveness* of a *learning opportunity* using known criteria (e.g., quality, continuity or efficiency measures).

Let's continue with the eastern Kentucky example. Suppose the mother had visited the emergency room on a given occasion and was taught how to use a thermometer (LO_1). Then, as reinforcement, she was asked about its use during a regular checkup in the physician's office (LO_2). This second learning opportunity would have provided important continuity to the first *LO*. Another possibility for continuity would have been to schedule a special followup visit with the educator in order to discuss any concerns the mother might then have about her child (LO_3). Each separate interaction can be identified as a discrete learning opportunity, the sum of which ($LO_1 + LO_2 + LO_3$) would serve to reinforce the mother's new learned behavior.

At the same time, each learning opportunity can be rated for its effectiveness. Although the initial visit to the emergency room might have been successful, it is possible that during other visits the mother might receive conflicting information, which would reduce the effectiveness of all the learning opportunities. Consequently, each learning opportunity requires review and rating in relation to its access, continuity, quality, and efficiency in order to determine its effectiveness. In turn, the overall effectiveness of the health education program is evaluated by examining the sum of the learning opportunities as well as their interaction.

The Distribution and Determinants of Health Education Programs

As a discipline, the field of health education is concerned with the distribution and determinants of learning opportunities that have to do with health and that occur in a given setting. Health educators want to determine where these learning opportunities might exist, what important variables are associated with their occurrence, and how they can be organized in order to maximize their potential for effecting health-related behavior and improved health.

A Model of a Health Education Delivery System

One way to illustrate how these issues can be addressed is to develop a paradigm that explains how we become "health educated." In Chapter 3 we developed a systems model to describe the delivery of health care services. In that model, which we will now apply to the delivery of health education (see Figure 5.1), there are inputs, processes, and outputs. There are variables within the health education system, variables outside the system that impact upon it, and a set of functions that measure the efficiency and effectiveness of the system. Inputs into this system of health education are people pursuing their own interests and seeking assistance from institutions in solving their problems. Their goal is to learn how to take care of themselves, their families, and their community; the means to accomplish this goal is the process of interacting with the health education delivery system. (For example, if a man has a disease or condition about which he is concerned, he might seek a physician who emphasizes teaching as part of the treatment, to learn what he can do to improve his health.) Other inputs into the system are all resources supporting the system of health education, including manpower, facilities, equipment, and financial support. All information and knowledge related to health or to a specific condition also become important inputs.

These inputs enter the health education system, defined as a set of learning opportunities distributed within a setting (or settings) at many different points. Each point represents a specific setting (site or location) for the potential provision of health education services (i.e., a learning opportunity). The following four variables are used to describe each point: (1) the learning opportunity is delivered in a geographic setting (e.g., a hospital, physician's office, or home); (2) the nature of the problem (the disease or condition) must be known, for it will determine the type of learning opportunity required; (3) the learning opportunity provided can be classified according to its level of prevention (primary, secondary, or tertiary); and, finally, (4) the structural characteristics of the learning opportunity can be defined (facility, organization, finance, manpower, and accountability).

As consumers enter the health education system—a set of learning opportunities distributed within a setting—or move from point to point, they may encounter difficulties or barriers that slow down or ultimately block their progress toward becoming health educated. To describe these barriers, we have labeled a set of variables as objectives: accessibility, quality,

Figure 5.1 *A Systems Model of Health Education Delivery*

External Constraints

Sociocultural forces
Economic forces
Technological forces
Political forces
Legal forces

Inputs

Individuals with needs
(lifestyles/biological)

Environmental factors
contributing to disease

Health resources available
(based upon constraints)

HEALTH EDUCATION
DELIVERY SYSTEM
(processes involving delivery
of health education)

Outputs (Outcomes)

Change in individuals' knowledge,
values, attitudes, practices

Change in institutions
(restructure the system)

Change in society
(restructure the society)

Health Education Service Points

Health Education System of
Planned Learning Opportunities

Objectives	Structural Features	Setting(s)	Type(s) of Service	Level of Prevention
Quality	Facility	Hospital	Medical	Primary
Continuity	Organization	Home	Social	Secondary
Efficiency	Finance	School	Wellness	Tertiary
Accessibility	Personnel	Voluntary organization	Nutritional	
	Accountability	Workplace	Occupational	
		Clinic	Mental/emotional	
		Health department	Etc.	

continuity, and efficiency. Consumers may also be affected by variables that exist outside of the system but that greatly influence how the health education system operates. This set of external constraints comprises socio-cultural, economic, technological, political, and legal forces.

Our model brings together the variety of perspectives needed to operationally define health education. It clearly distinguishes among structure, process, and outcomes. From a structural perspective, it is clear that if a learning opportunity is to occur, it must be organized and have its resources within the setting. Further, although each learning opportunity is a discrete entity with its own features, it is obvious that we must be concerned with the interaction of all possible learning opportunities and how they relate to each other if we are to provide reinforcement and expanded opportunities for learning. Last, the model helps to define those areas targeted for change by health educators, including changes in individual behaviors and lifestyles, changes in an institution's behavior, and changes in a society's ways of behaving. We have called these changes outcomes of health education practice.

Objectives for Health Education Practice

We can now use our model to develop detailed objectives for a health education practice. Specifically, our objectives are to provide health education services (1) that are accessible to consumers, (2) that are of high quality, (3) that assure consumers a continuing relationship with educators until their needs are met, and (4) that are efficient and assure the economical use of health resources.

Accessibility.   How do we make it possible for individuals to gain access to health education services? First, we must provide individuals with the opportunity to obtain these services when they enter an agency or institution offering such services. For example, courses in school health should be available for all children enrolled in the public schools. Patients entering the medical care system should have available to them health education services relevant to their illness, and employees in a factory should have available health education materials relevant to their health and safety at work. Second, we must also provide a wide range of health education services in the community, that is, in a variety of settings, including medical care facilities, schools, and worksites. Achieving this objective requires not only the training and employment of health educators but also the readiness of community agencies to offer these services. Third, we should provide enough health education services so that health professionals can refer consumers to these services with the expectation that there are sufficient services available to meet consumer needs.

Quality.   The assurance of high-quality educational services to consumers depends on several factors. These factors include the level of training of health educators, the continuous evaluation of the effectiveness of health education programs, and open communication between health educators and consumers about consumer satisfaction or dissatisfaction with the programs in which they have participated.

Continuity.   This objective is based on the assumption that the prevention of illness is a continuous activity and that, therefore, health education services ought to be available to consumers throughout their lives. To achieve this objective, communities should offer health education services that are both planned and coordinated. For example, centralized health education planning would effectively coordinate the health education services of various community agencies such as health maintenance organizations, school medical care facilities, and so on.

Efficiency.   Assuring this objective requires adequate financing of health education services as well as efficient administration of these services. Currently the overwhelming percentage of funding for health care goes for the medical care of those already ill. A commitment to the prevention of illness requires that public policy decisions on the financing of health care shift some of the money now allotted to medical care to health education services. All societies face the competing claims of various services for a limited amount of resources. Prevention of illness is a major justification for the public to provide resources for health education services. Health educators, however, are expected to use those resources in an effective and cost-efficient manner.

Elements of Health Education Practice

The model we have used to describe the distribution and determinants of health education services can also help us to understand and explain the evolving practice of health education. At this point it should be clear that any given health educator works within a setting (or settings), and utilizes skills that are appropriate to these settings, to bring about desired outcomes. Consequently, to fully understand health education practice we need to further examine these three fundamental elements of settings, outcomes, and skills. To help explain these relationships and place them into context, we have developed an additional paradigm, shown in Figure 5.2 (see p. 104).

Settings

For our purposes, a setting is where a health education program exists and where the consumer is presented with learning opportunities. Each

Figure 5.2   *Interrelationships of Skills, Settings, and Outcomes in Health Education Practice*

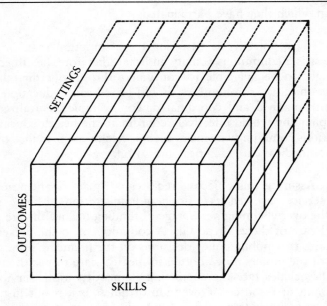

Source: This model was originally developed by Elena Sliepcevich, Alan Henderson, and Ira J. Bates (1976).

setting can be divided into subunits that constitute the "health education service points," where learning opportunities occur. For example, Mary H. works for the state heart association (a setting) and helps to organize cardiopulmonary resuscitation (CPR) classes at the local YMCA (a service point within a setting). A setting is described by the following structural characteristics: (1) where it is located (which we have called *facility* in our model); (2) how it is organized; (3) how it is financed; (4) which personnel provide the health education services; and (5) to whom it is accountable or responsible.

From a myriad of possible settings, we can generalize six categories of settings in which health education specialists are currently employed. These include

   1. Primary-care settings: Ambulatory clinics where medical and dental services are provided to general populations
   2. Health maintenance organizations: Prepaid group practice organizations designed to meet the total health needs of certain populations

3. Hospitals and other clinical settings: Hospitals or ambulatory clinics, and other providers of direct health services
4. School and academic settings: Elementary, middle, junior, and senior high schools; colleges and universities; and continuing education and adult education programs
5. Occupational health settings: Unions, industries, and other workplace-oriented settings
6. Community health settings: Public health agencies at local, state, and federal government levels, as well as voluntary, categorical-disease-based agencies such as heart associations and lung associations, or geographic-centered agencies such as regional health systems agencies

It is important to note that all of these settings are interrelated and open-ended. Our model has been designed to be flexible and adaptable in order to adjust to changes in health and education and in those settings where health educators continue to practice.

Outcomes

A second element, equally important in understanding health education practice, is the desired outcome or end result of health education programs. Actual outcomes that health educators would be able to effect depend largely on the particular setting and the range of skills that are required to plan and conduct health education within that particular setting. These outcomes are, for the most part, determined by the organizational goals of the setting. Essential requirements are the ability to specify desired outcomes and the capacity to plan, organize, operate, and evaluate the educational programs that will bring about these outcomes. An appropriately trained health educator will possess those skills necessary to effect desired outcomes as defined by a given setting.

Skills

The third element needed to comprehend the practice of health education involves the range and types of skills that health educators apply in the setting in which they are employed. It is crucial for professional health educators to develop skills that are both flexible and adaptable in their application and function to the setting. Sliepcevich (1975) has developed a core of eight skills that meet these requirements. Health educators must be skilled in

1. Learning and behavioral theory
2. Communication
3. Process and methods
4. Knowledge and resources

5. Research and evaluation
6. Planning and policy formation
7. Organization and administration
8. Coordination and supervision

These eight skill areas are interrelated and interdependent; they are an integral part of the functions of health educators in a specific setting. Although we have discussed settings, outcomes, and skills as separate elements, in practice they should not be separated. The setting, to a degree, determines the outcome, which in turn, determines the skills required by the setting. For example, we know from experience that academic settings require the health educators they employ to focus largely on first- and second-order micro changes as outcomes. Using our model, we can ask, Which learning or behavioral theories are appropriate for this setting? Conversely, if we are interested in creating a given outcome, there are certain settings that will more likely allow the desired outcome of micro change to be realized.

In order to understand the conceptual framework of settings, skills, and outcomes and their interrelationships, Chapters 6, 7, and 8 will deal directly with these components of our model. Chapter 6 describes settings for practice and how health educators function within a given environment. Chapter 7 identifies those competencies needed for practice and Chapter 8 focuses upon health education outcomes.

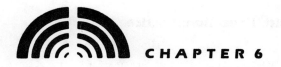

CHAPTER 6

Health Education Programs: Settings for Practice

Historically, health educators have been viewed as practicing in two specific kinds of settings: the community, usually defined by some geographic boundary, and educational institutions, usually elementary and secondary schools. Typically, community health was administered from the county or city public health agency that had the responsibility for public health within the county in which the agency was located. Community health education was one aspect of public health practice, and its development paralleled that of other public health programs. (We will more closely examine the evolution of community health education in public health settings in Chapter 10.)

Health education in the schools evolved with concern over physical fitness and education in public schools. In the 1950's, as compulsory public education spread throughout the country, health education in school settings became a separate and distinct field from physical education. Separate university courses prepared health educators for work in school settings, with some preparation for community health programs included. Public health education became formalized as part of the curriculum within schools of public health concerned with preparing public health professionals. Some school health education courses were found within these professional schools. In most instances, concepts of health education in both school and public health settings evolved in a parallel fashion.

Current Settings for Health Education Practice

The School Health Setting

Schools can be viewed as educational settings in which health educators have opportunities to provide a wide range of health education to the nation's children. These learning opportunities may take place in a human sexuality class, for instance, or while a student visits the nurse's office or reviews the week's menus for the school cafeteria. The basic idea behind school health education is that informed children become informed adults: health-educated people who are more likely to have an increased capacity for self-care and intelligent decision making about their use of the health care system and about public health policy. Despite the potential of the school setting, school districts have been slow to make use of the opportunities available. School health education programs have suffered from a multitude of problems, such as low priority in the school system, the narrowness of "acceptable" content, a shortage of trained health education teachers, and constraints resulting from outside community pressure.

Accelerated social forces have had a strong impact on the development of school health education. No longer can the school setting be characterized in a singular manner. Rather, it must be viewed with multiplicity. For example, what preparation is required for a health educator to work in an elementary school today? Is the school located in a coal-mining town? In a rural agricultural community? In an inner-city ghetto? Is there a need for health education in vocational and technical schools? What are the health education needs of special populations, such as vision- and hearing-impaired individuals? The field of health education has experienced rapid changes in response to the needs of these different types of schools.

Because of the social forces within which school health education exists, changes in the school health setting have not always been positive. Education as a social institution is subject to the same forces that affect other segments of society. In 1971, for instance, the Illinois legislature passed the Critical Health Problems and Comprehensive Health Education Act, requiring that health be taught in schools by certified teachers. It has yet to be implemented. Instead, many of the positions for which current undergraduates compete will be filled by people already in the teaching profession who have upgraded their skills to an acceptable level. Moreover, the Illinois Office of Education projects that state public school enrollments will decline from 2,373,659 in 1971 to between 1,889,000 and 1,996,000 in 1985, producing both a similarly declining enrollment at colleges and universities and declining needs for teacher preparation. In 1974 the Illinois Office of Education noted that "if present pupil-teacher ratios were maintained there would be a need for eleven to twenty thousand fewer teachers by 1985." The Office of Education further noted that of the 12,000 teachers needed each year in the state, nearly 40 percent are teachers reentering the educational arena. Only the balance of 5,900 to 7,300 positions will be available for newly credentialed teachers. Yet in 1973 13,247 prospective new teachers graduated.

The Community Health Setting

The goals of community health education programs are disease prevention, health promotion, and health protection within the context of a "community." The aim of such programs is to identify individuals at risk, make them conscious of that risk, and provide an education program that will help them reduce it. Community health education programs generally serve large populations, which can usually be defined by a geographical or functional unit. The geographical unit normally falls within an established political boundary. The functional unit is composed of individuals who share some common characteristic (such as socioeconomic level, ethnic origin, age, or religious affiliation) that is used to define the community.

Rothman (1968) has identified three models of community health education practice. He calls these models locality development, social planning, and social action. The locality, or community, development model strives for education for participative membership and shared decision making as its primary goal. In contrast, the focus of the social-planning approach is task-oriented, toward solving community problems. For example, social-planning organizations—such as mental health departments, urban renewal authorities, and commissions on alcoholism—are often mandated to deal with concrete social problems. The third approach, social action, is primarily concerned with establishing local-based power and decision-making centers within the community. This approach was used in the 1960's, for example, when the Office of Economic Opportunity set up programs designed to increase citizen participation in public policymaking. Poor people were trained to organize themselves to influence governmental decisions that affected their living conditions.

Other settings for the practice of community health education are voluntary health agencies at the local, state, and national levels. There are presently about 70 national health agencies affiliated with the National Health Council, the majority of which are engaged in some practice of health education. Generally, these programs are designed to increase public awareness about important health problems. Examples are the American Cancer Society, which is well known for its campaign to educate the public to the seven danger signals for cancer, the American Heart Association, the Planned Parenthood Federation of America, and the National Safety Council.

Just as with our past concepts of schools, past ideas of communities have been restricted to geographical or political definitions. The terms *city, county,* and *state* have been used synonymously with *community*. Community health sites have been further constrained by limiting definitions to health departments (e.g., local, county, or state) or voluntary agencies (e.g., cancer, heart, lung). As Bowman (1976) has found, however, the traditional concept of community is not obsolete. Public health educators have moved into a number of nontraditional settings, with the result that "the number of choices for practice open to public health educators at present is far greater than at any time in the history of the profession" (Bowman, 1976, p. 243). Another result has been "problems for the profession in defining its mission and relative role and status among other health professionals"; yet Bowman foresees an encouraging outcome:

> As a final comment, one might point out that the specific roles and functions in such emerging settings as patient education, manpower training and continuing education, health education for preschool children and their parents, self-instruction, health communications programs, and others will place greater stress on the analysis of learning tasks, behavioral learning objectives, instructional methodology to achieve specific learning goals, and the evaluation of learning. Thus it appears that the roles and functions of public health educators in the future may become more truly those of teachers, instructors, educators —perhaps more so than at any time since the effective separation of school health and public health education as independent professional fields.

The developments Bowman discusses have effectively served to broaden the concept of community for health education to include (1) areas where people of similar or varying age groups and backgrounds congregate for a specific purpose and (2) settings in which people are found for brief or extended periods of time and that provide situations in which education is feasible. In these settings, the population, at a given time, is likely to be motivated or health oriented for a variety of reasons. Thus, an individual may move from one "community" to another in a given day or period of time. When viewed in this manner, communities become interdependent and interrelated. The entire life cycle of the individual, family, and community is encompassed within this perspective.

Other Settings for Health Education Practice

Existing settings for health education practice have been expanded and refined while new settings have been added. For example, hospitals and outpatient clinics now employ health education specialists to provide patients with educational opportunities as well as outreach and follow-up services. These positions, frequently referred to as "health education coordinators," have provided an emerging role for health education practice.

Clinical health care settings are organized to serve patients. Consumers become patients when they recognize a health problem and seek out a physician, clinic, hospital or some other health care provider or institution. Patient education in these settings is generally concerned with patient compliance with, or adherence to, therapeutic regimens. Patients' refusal to accept therapeutic regimens is well documented. Recent studies indicate that about one-third never comply, one-third always comply, and one-third sometimes comply (Haynes, 1979).

Although health education in clinical settings has expanded, many health educators are concerned about the emphasis on "compliance," since it seems to reflect a specific provider-patient model that places the provider in the role of authority and the patient in the role of submissiveness. As we have suggested, there are other models of provider-patient relationships (i.e., the teaching of theories and principles) that are more in keeping with the democratic methods exemplified by Mayhew Derryberry, Dorothy Nyswander, and other pioneers of health education.

Other settings for health education practice are found in those agencies that mandate the involvement of consumers in decision making about health policy. For example, individuals are often exposed to occupational hazards at their places of work. These people have a unique opportunity to identify potential hazards and reduce their risk of disease occurrence. The education of workers at all levels of the work place is referred to as occupational health education.

In recent years the Occupational Safety and Health Administration (OSHA) organized extensive employee education programs so that employees may both identify health hazards in their work environment and prevent injuries to themselves because of unsafe acts. The OSHA identified two categories that place workers at risk: (1) the presence of safety hazards or dangerous physical conditions such as inadequate guards on machinery, and (2) the existence of health hazards such as unsafe levels of toxic substances or harmful physical agents such as carbon monoxide and asbestos. In addition, stress has recently been recognized as an occupational hazard. Findings in Great Britain (1981), for example, show that more work hours are lost through stress-related mental and emotional problems than through physical injuries. It is anticipated that the rising costs of medical insurance, paid by industry, will make it cost-efficient for industry to develop occupational health education programs. At the same time, decreasing federal support for these programs may compound the overall problem.

Additional settings that employ health education specialists are agencies involved in training (especially for allied health personnel and continuing programs for all health personnel) and categorical programs, such as gerontological, ecological, environmental, child development, family planning, health insurance marketing, and rural cooperative extension services. Still other health educators deal with educational technology such as instructional media or health communications.

Figure 6.1 *Objectives and Dimensions of Health Education Systems*

Objectives of a Health System	Dimensions of Program Plans				
	Facility	Organization	Finance	Personnel	Accountability
Access					
Quality					
Continuity					
Efficiency					

Characteristics of Health Education Settings

In order to better understand relationships between settings and outcomes for health education practice, as described in Chapter 5, Figure 5.2, it is important for us now to review in detail the characteristics of settings. In our previous discussion of a health education program, we identified four major objectives, or criteria of effectiveness, of health education programs: accessibility, quality, continuity, and efficiency. In addition, we suggested that five structural features, or dimensions, of settings were directly related to outcomes. These were facility, organization, finance, personnel, and accountability. We have used these variables to develop the matrix shown in Figure 6.1.

Five Dimensions of Settings

The important point about these five dimensions is that they determine whether a health education program can function in a particular setting; that is, they act as major determinants of both the number and effectiveness of the learning opportunities that can occur in a given setting. To explain the use of this matrix, let's look at some examples. First, we'll return to the case of the mother with the sick child in eastern Kentucky, which we discussed earlier, in Chapter 5. We'll begin by looking at where the initial learning opportunity occurred in that setting, remembering that an ideal learning opportunity offers the greatest potential for learning about health and is directly related to the setting in which it occurs. In our Kentucky example the time variable was crucial because of the motivating influence brought about by the immediacy of the situation. Thus the learning opportunity with the most potential (as determined by this setting) immediately followed the crisis, in the emergency room.

In order for that "teachable moment" to happen, it was necessary that there be a quiet place (facility), with appropriately trained staff members (personnel), prepared to teach the mother (organization). In addition to having time available to teach, the educator would need to be paid for these services (finance), and be responsible to someone for performing them (accountability). As we can more clearly see by applying this specific information to our matrix, there are a number of reasons why this particular approach to teaching and learning might be difficult to implement within an emergency room setting. An emergency room is not ordinarily an efficient facility in which to teach because of the nature of its intended purpose for use by the critically ill and the injured. The organization of a deliberate, planned educational intervention would be crucial in this setting.

The following case study, reported in the Springfield, Massachusetts, *Valley Advocate* (July 1, 1981), illustrates the five determinants in a different setting.

Sex Ed Tools

Kathryn Bosch has been foraging. So far, her collection includes these slogans:

Get nailed by a carpenter. I like sex. Let's make it tonight. You'd smile too if you'd just been laid. Bankers do it with interest . . . with penalty for early withdrawal. Firemen are always in heat. Give it to me one more time. Once a week is not enough. Make it in Massachusetts.

Bumper stickers, buttons, song lyrics. Advertisements, not from girlie mags, but from *Good Housekeeping, Seventeen, Readers Digest,* and *The New York Times.*

Bosch's purpose in collecting these media blurbs is not to start a new specialty shop. Rather, as Community Health Educator for the Family Planning Council of Western Massachusetts, she has assembled such messages into a slide-tape presentation. Her show is designed to convince parents of adolescents and pre-adolescents that their children are constantly assaulted with sexual innuendoes that scream, "Do it!" What kids need, she insists, is instruction in self-worth, self-understanding, communication of feelings as well as a knowledge of physiology and anatomy. She calls this approach "sexuality education" and encourages parents, churches and schools to provide it.

Contrary to parents' forebodings, sexuality education programs encourage teenagers to exercise restraint: to feel able to resist peer pressure and, if they decide to become sexually active, to use birth control. The programs aim to counter the rash of teenage pregnancies, now up to one million nationwide.

Sexuality education programs are not widespread in this area, despite the efforts of Bosch and others. Smith School in Northampton started one for 10- and 11-year-olds this past year; Mahar Regional High School in Orange has a two-week family life program for seventh graders as part of the science curriculum that is now in its third year; Bement School in Old Deerfield has courses for seventh, eighth and ninth graders and parents. Many other communities, such as Easthampton, have nothing. With Proposition 2½, even schools like Northampton High School, which favor inclusion of such programs in the curriculum, are cutting back due to lack of funds.

Yet, after long spells of controversy, and even with financial restraints, new programs are popping up here and there. Amherst recently initiated a course for eighth graders that will begin in the fall. Several churches, including Edwards Church in Northampton, have been receptive to the idea.

Bosch showed her slide-tape for the first time in a four-week series for parents at Bay State Medical Center in Springfield. Amidst gasps, nervous giggles, and "oh, no's," she explained the family planning council's perspective: Sexual information is bombarding young people continually. To keep them away from it, kids would have to be locked in closets. Do parents want advertisements and other profit-governed teasers to be the sole source of their children's learning about sex? Or will they support classes taught by responsible adults?

Randy Ring

In this case, Kathryn Bosch, the health educator, has two major concerns: first, to expand the capacity of school settings to provide an increased number of learning opportunities for teenagers and, second, to increase the effectiveness of current sexuality education programs. Bosch's anticipated outcome for both these efforts is that teenagers would be better able to make informed choices concerning their own sexuality, thereby changing their sexual behavior and lifestyles. From a macro perspective, she is concerned with changing school systems.

Several important points can be made about this case. Bosch recognizes that teenagers are already exposed to a number of learning opportunities in their social environment. She acknowledges that there are significant social forces that have a negative impact on teenage behavior. Next, she defines her task as identifying these forces and bringing them into public awareness, particularly to those parents with teenage sons and daughters. To effect the outcome she has determined (i.e., to provide teenagers with opportunities and skills to make informed choices), she is prepared to engage in first-order macro change. She wants to change school systems' current programs.

Referring to the matrix, we can ask questions that are appropriate to this case:

Where and when do students go to school? (facility)

What current learning opportunities in sex education exist in the school system? (organization)

Who teaches these courses? What are their credentials? (personnel)

How are these courses currently financed or supported? (finance)

To whom is the teacher accountable for content and process of sexuality education programs? (accountability)

Are the curriculum content, resources, and materials adequate? (organization)

Are the content and process acceptable to students? to parents? to the community at large? (accountability)

What is the continuity of the learning opportunities as they occur within the grade levels? (organization)

Is there a central source of information for students? parents? teachers? (organization)

As we learned in Chapter 4, one of the most basic questions health educators must ask is, What do we want to change? Obviously the answer will be as different as are the constraints placed on each setting. Targets for change in this case could include teenagers' behavior, their lifestyles, institutions that directly affect their behaviors and lifestyles, and those societal forces that have conspired to make teenagers uninformed regarding their sexuality.

The setting in which Bosch is employed is not organized or financed in such a way as to directly change widespread social forces. The limitations of this setting prohibit, to a large degree, direct public confrontation on these issues. For example, Bosch would have no legal power to have *Playboy* magazine removed from the racks of newstands. (Nor would a health educator who is concerned with voluntary, informed decision making support such an effort.) Alternatively, for this agency, to provide direct educational services to teenagers (i.e., micro change) would be very inefficient and cost prohibitive. We are thus left with the institutional-change approach of the school setting which appears to be the most effective way to maximize learning opportunities about sexuality.

The Impact of Societal Values on Settings

In Chapter 4, we raised the issue of the effect of societies' social values on the health educator's options to create change. We now return to this issue from the perspective that institutions (settings), because of the way they are organized, reflect the beliefs, values, and norms of the society that they serve. Health educators cannot function independently of these settings. At the same time, it is these very institutions that are the targets for change. Society often limits the scope of an institution's activities or functions to specifically defined areas. If health educators want to create change within a setting, then they must understand the societal forces that affect that setting and also recognize how these forces place boundaries around its functions. To illustrate this point, let's continue with the example of the health education program in the rural clinic in eastern Kentucky.

Patient education is an essential element in the clinic's approach to health care. Most of the chronic problems seen at the clinic—obesity, hypertension, diabetes, chronic pulmonary disease—require patient cooperation for optimum management. It has taken a while for the clinic staff to convince patients, raised to see fatness as a sign of health and beauty, that obesity is unhealthy and unattractive. The message seems to have gotten across. When several nurses began a weekly obesity class last January, they were stunned to find that more than 80 people had enrolled.

The clinic staff also has concentrated on improving pre- and postnatal care. Child care classes are scheduled for women in their last few months of pregnancy. To encourage them and their husbands to attend, the clinic offers a reduction in obstetric fees of $5 for each class the mother attends, with another $5 off for each class the father attends. A week after a new mother brings her infant home from the hospital, a nurse from the clinic visits them at home to respond to questions and to observe the child's surroundings. One nurse, Jan Stumbo recalls, found that a new mother was keeping her baby's bottle in the creek because the family had no refrigerator, and the insufficiently cooled milk was giving the infant constant diarrhea.

The lack of some of the modern amenities that we take for granted —refrigeration, plumbing, heating—creates certain health problems that the clinic cannot solve. Other health problems are the result of years of poverty, poor nutrition, and dismal working conditions in the mines. But if the clinic cannot make the mountain people healthier, it can help them achieve what Bailey calls their "health potential" and help improve the length and quality of lives that must remain something less than ideal (Henig, 1976, pp. 24–27).

In this case the clinic's scope (or defined area of responsibility) was limited by societal forces within the culture to the provision of "medical care." To address the basic problems underlying the existing health conditions—poverty, poor nutrition, dismal working conditions in coal mines— would mean addressing social and economic forces that require second-order macro change. In this setting, such change was unlikely to occur because of the impact of society's values upon the setting. Recognition of this by the clinic staff is reflected in Henig's statement that the clinic cannot solve these problems—that it simply is not within the scope of the clinic to attempt to produce second-order macro change).

Another illustration of this point can be found in the following case study in an international setting. Nigerian Brain Fatigue Syndrome (NBFS) is a name given to a set of conditions associated with Nigerian students attending westernized school systems (both in Nigeria and other countries). The clinical profile of the syndrome includes headaches, vision problems, and an inability to sleep, concentrate, or retain information. Drug use is associated with the syndrome, particularly of marijuana and amphetamines. The symptoms are most likely to occur during times of academic stress, notably during comprehensive exams. (Such symptoms are not unlike those experienced by American students during finals week.)

Health officials of the Nigerian government view the condition as a psychiatric problem, and students presenting complaints are referred for psychiatric treatment. In Nigeria, however, strong social stigmas are associated with any type of psychiatric treatment. Students view the problem as a "spell" cast upon them by other, competing students. Their preferred mode of treatment is the traditional healer, in this case a witch doctor, who is believed to have the power to remove the spell or cast other spells.

Jay Scott was on assignment from the Agency for International Development in Nigeria for two years. He was asked by the Nigerian Ministry of Health to investigate the problem and advise the government. After studying the problem, Scott concluded that current approaches to psychiatric treatment of the syndrome were ineffective. He explained that, for a variety of reasons, Nigerian students reject both referral and treatment; the result is an exacerbation of the problem. Scott explained that the students behaved as they did, in part, because the "psychiatric labels" placed upon them, after they accepted the psychiatric treatment modality, remained with them throughout their lives and, in some instances, prohibited their employment in certain positions. Moreover, their cultural belief system, which accepted supernatural explanations of illnesses, did not recognize "western, technological medicine" as a solution to their problem.

There were two approaches to resolving this problem. One approach was to integrate the traditional healer into the existing psychiatric system (i.e., first-order macro change). The second approach involved addressing the external social forces that were identified as having initially created the problem (second-order macro change). The key to both approaches was in understanding the Nigerian culture. Nigerian children are taught to work together within family structures and tribes. They are taught to function, think, and behave from the perspective of group cooperation. When they enter a westernized school system, which is largely based on individual (rather than group) accomplishment, and on competition at all levels, their values are in conflict with the setting. To deal with this problem of "disjointedness," Nigerian students frequently invoke their supernatural beliefs. Interestingly, this mode of adaptation in response to school-related stress is not uncommon in American cultures (e.g., wearing a "lucky" shirt on test day; the use of alcohol and drugs or prayer and meditation).

Nigerian government officials, desiring to modernize their country, have rejected the traditional healer as part of their treatment system, believing that such practices have no place in a "developed" country. For Scott, the problem lacked a workable solution in the short term. In this setting, as an international consultant, his task was one of developing strategies that would influence leaders in the Ministry of Health to recognize the conflicting values that were at the root of the problem. Although he might have engaged in second-order macro change in this setting, he could not have directly instituted policies that would have changed either the Nigerian health system or the manner in which Nigerian school systems operated.

The three examples we've examined illustrate the direct relationship between a setting and the environment in which it exists. The existence of poverty as an unfortunate part of life for the clients of the Kentucky clinic served to shape the boundaries of the health educators' interventions. In our Massachusetts example, although removal of media influences that create pressure on teenagers to express their sexual behaviors may have been ideal, Kathryn Bosch's agency was limited in its direct action because of other societal values. For Jay Scott, the Nigerian culture, a blend of traditional and modern beliefs and practices, required a clear understanding of both. Thus health educators, working in any setting, must understand the external environment and its components, particularly the beliefs, values, and norms of that environment. This environment is the source of powerful social forces that define the scope of the setting in which health educators must function.

Just as the environment shapes the setting, the setting in turn determines those skills that are necessary for health educators to be effective. In Chapter 7 we will explore eight skill areas in which health educators must be competent.

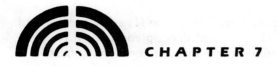

CHAPTER 7

Health Education Programs: Skills for Practice

What skills are needed to practice health education? Is there a relationship between settings and skills? What is the difference between the health education process and a health education program? What are the skills necessary to practice in a community health agency setting? In a school setting? What are the differences between the skills required in a school health education setting and a voluntary health setting?

To answer these questions, we first need to restate our operational definition of health education. Health education is a deliberate, planned intervention that occurs in a setting at a given point in time and involves an interaction between teacher and learner. In this chapter, we will (1) identify the necessary competencies that distinguish health educators from professionals in other health disciplines. We will then (2) delineate the specific skills necessary for practice, (3) develop a model for health education planning and evaluation that outlines, step by step, how health education is practiced in any setting, and (4) examine health education practice in detail, illustrating linkages between theory and practice and variations in skill requirements for different settings.

The Essential Competencies of a Health Educator

Health educators are people who, working within a given setting, possess certain skills in educational processes that enable them to effect specific changes (outcomes) which, in turn affect health status. Five competencies distinguish health educators from professionals in other health disciplines. Health educators must be able to (1) assess the needs of settings for health education, (2) plan and develop educational interventions, (3) implement those interventions through the development of a health education program, (4) evaluate the program, and (5) work with people in the process. Taken together, these five competencies provide the health educator with the ability to enter a given setting and provide an effective educational intervention.

Assessing a Given Setting

A health educator must be able to assess a given setting, within the context of its environment, in order to determine what needs to be changed. In other words, a health educator must be able to identify those outcomes that could potentially affect health status and that could be accomplished within that setting (i.e., are appropriate for the setting). This essential competency—the ability to conduct a needs assessment of a setting—is basic to the practice of health education. Health educators must be able to understand how a setting functions in relation to its environment and how activities that occur in the setting may affect health status.

Social forces within the external environment define a setting (or institution), which, in turn, is structured to provide services to help people with their needs. Consequently, the society defines, to a large extent, the setting's scope and the approaches that are considered acceptable for meeting these needs. For example, we don't learn to play a piano in a hospital; nor do we go to the teacher for treatment of a broken leg.

At the same time, a setting defines peoples' needs by specifying the constituency it serves and the interventions that are most appropriate for meeting the needs of that constituency. These interventions define the specific outcomes (i.e., changes that affect health status) about which the setting is concerned. A health educator must understand these relationships in order to determine what needs to be changed and what outcomes are appropriate for a specific setting. In our eastern Kentucky example (introduced in Chapter 5), society limited the scope of the rural health clinic to treatment of mountain people with "medical problems." The clinic's interventions involved diagnosis and treatment of illnesses. An important part of the treatment was changing peoples' behaviors (first-order micro change) and, to a limited extent, lifestyles (second-order micro change). The nature of the setting did not permit health educators to define what needed to be changed as a lack of money or a lack of employment opportunities; consequently, it was not possible for the health educators to engage in second-order macro change. (It should be noted that health educators did accomplish first-order macro change within the clinic itself by establishing patient education programs where they did not previously exist).

The important point for health education practice is that, by their very nature, specific settings have specific outcomes that necessitate specific skills for the health educator. Although these skills are generally similar, the combination or mix will be quite different in varying settings.

Planning and Developing Educational Interventions

The second competency a health educator must possess is the ability to plan and develop educational interventions, within the context of a given setting, that will produce specific outcomes (changes that affect health status). Health educators must be able to identify the points at which learning opportunities occur within a setting and be able to assess their potential effectiveness as planned educational interventions.

In the design of educational programs, health educators are concerned with the distribution of learning opportunities and how each can be maximized to effect a specific outcome. In this sense, health educators seek both to increase the number of learning opportunities by expanding the capacity of the setting to provide them and to improve the effectiveness of the current opportunities by evaluating their accessibility, quality, continuity, and efficiency. In developing planned interventions, health educators must be able to specify why the educational intervention is needed. What is its purpose? For whom is it intended? When, and where, is the program to occur? Who will provide the teaching? What methods will be used? Are they appropriate? How will the program be evaluated? In essence, health educators are preparing a written description of those variables that together constitute an educational intervention: need, objectives, methods, evaluation, and, of course, the learner.

Implementing Planned Educational Programs

The third essential competency of a health educator is the ability to organize and carry out these planned educational interventions. The plan is a description of a proposed action that the health educator follows, in a series of specific steps, to test the worth and usefulness of the intervention. To organize and implement the plan, it is first necessary to structure a demonstration, which initially serves to validate the plan and also provides useful information regarding the amount of resources (facilities, budget, personnel, materials) needed to begin a full-scale operation. Once the full-scale operation is underway, the health educator must then manage the program—prepare a budget, monitor expenditures, write job descriptions, delegate responsibility, hire personnel, and evaluate performance.

Evaluating Health Education Programs

The fourth necessary competency of a health educator is the ability to evaluate a health education program. The term *evaluate* means to place value upon, using selected criteria. Evaluation occurs at a variety of levels and serves several purposes. Health educators need to evaluate (1) research in the preparation of a plan, (2) alternative plans, in the preparation of a demonstration, (3) several demonstrations, in the validation of a program, and (4) a program in terms of its impact on the need identified by the plan. Evaluation serves several purposes. It can enhance health education practice by further clarifying "what health education can or cannot do, or by validating which methods are effective" (APHA, 1978). As such, it provides a stronger base for practice. Evaluation also enables health educators to measure the success of a program for policymakers such as government officials or legislators.

Working with People

Finally, the fifth, and most essential, competency of a health educator is the ability to work with people in the totality of the process. As Derryberry (1952) noted in a classic explanation, "The importance of good human relations for any learning situation can hardly be overestimated. This involves 'acceptance' of other people, no matter who or what they are; respect for personality; and a friendly approach based on an innate inclination to like and work with people" (p. 2). The crucial difference, however, between a health educator and someone involved in any other health discipline lies in the word *totality* in our definition. A health educator is involved with a variety of people throughout a multistage process of assessing a given setting, planning and developing educational interventions, organizing and carrying out programs, and evaluating those programs.

Principally, the role of a health educator in these activities is that of facilitator among providers, consumers, administrators, interest groups, and others who desire change. They seek to change their own behavior, other peoples' behaviors, the "system," or society itself. The health educator becomes the pivotal point for bringing about those actions necessary for change.

Skills for Health Education Practice

In Chapter 5, we introduced a model of health education practice that identified eight interrelated and interdependent skills fundamental to the practice of health education. Now, as we examine the practice of health education more closely, we'll see that health professionals must be skilled in (1) learning and behavioral theory, (2) communication, (3) process and methods, (4) knowledge and resources, (5) research and evaluation, (6) planning and policy formulation, (7) organization and administration, and (8) coordination and supervision.

Learning and Behavioral Theory

Health education is similar to general education in that it is concerned with changes in the knowledge, attitudes, and behavior of people. Its purpose is to develop health practices that are believed to bring about the best possible state of individual well being. In order for health education to be effective, its planning, methods, and procedures must take into consideration not only the processes by which people acquire knowledge, change their attitudes, and modify their behavior, but also the factors that influence such changes.

Because, more than anything else, the role of the health educator is that of teacher, competency in behavioral and educational theory is essential to the practice. Health educators must be able to answer those questions that encompass behavioral theory (How do we explain a person's, group's, or society's behavior?). They want to know, moreover, not only how to understand behavior but how to change the behaviors of persons, groups, or societies. The fundamental difference between the practice of health education and other behavioral sciences is that, while we wish to change or modify other peoples' behaviors, the strategies employed embody educational principles. Therefore, they are voluntary and democratic, and give the learner control over choices.

From this perspective, the health educator is interested in how we learn. Why do we learn? When do we learn? Where do we learn? Who is most likely to learn? And similarly, How do we teach? Why do we teach? When do we teach? As the American Public Health Association Policy Statement makes clear, "Health education is more than the provision of information. While health education includes acquiring knowledge about health matters, its purpose is the use of that knowledge. It addresses the formation of values, the acquisition of decision-making skills and the adoption of reinforcement of desirable health practices. Health education honors individuals' right to privacy, their right to meaningful information, and their right to make their own choices" (APHA, 1978, p. 2).

Communication

To know how to communicate effectively, health educators must first be aware of their audience (i.e., the learner). Audiences—targets for change—will vary according to their culture, maturation, motivation, and needs. Accordingly, methods of communication will also vary. For example, a film containing specific details about how to take care of a chronic illness would be inappropriate for second graders. A brochure explaining a hospitals' services would be ineffective in a Hispanic community if it were written in English.

Health educators utilize interpersonal and group communications, as well as mass media, in their practice. They need to be able to answer the following questions: What are the ways in which we communicate with other people? How do we describe a particular sender-receiver relationship? How do we avoid the interference of "static" in communications? What are the criteria for selecting appropriate modes of communication (e.g., oral—personal, small groups, or electronic media—versus written—pamphlets, advertisements, newspapers, handbooks—and so forth)?

Process and Methods

An old proverb says that if you give a man a fish, he will eat for a day, but if you teach him to fish, he will feed the world. In the same manner, the health education process involves teaching people to care for themselves, their families, and their communities, and improve all their lives.

Health educators are often not the primary teachers, however. They are, in essence, the teacher's teacher. In other words, the health educator frequently does not present the primary learning opportunity to the receiver but, instead, is responsible for the initiation and management of these opportunities. The health educator probably spends more time teaching others how to teach than participating in a traditional teacher-student role.

Just as communication theory forms a basis for part of health education practice, theories about process and methods must also be understood and applied by health educators. As the APHA Policy Statement explains, "since no single method can be expected to be effective with all persons under all circumstances, . . . the implementation of a health education program requires the use of a variety of methods." Indeed, "a combination of methods organized in a systems approach is more likely to achieve a desired result" (1978, p. 2). According to Ross and Mico (1980), a health educator's inventory of methods might include "group facilitation, nominal group technique, role clarification, role playing, 3d party intervention and arbitration, constructive confrontation, consultation, memorandum of agreement, mass communication, conference method, meetings, simulation, case method, coaching, interviewing, lectures, personal instruction, and programmed instruction" (pp. 214–215).

Certainly a familiarity with each of these methods is useful for the health educator, but it is not the determining factor. What a health educator must know is which process and methods will create a desired outcome in a given setting.

Knowledge and Resources

If one is going to teach anything, one must have access to a base of knowledge that forms the content of the instruction. This content primarily comprises those theories and principles we wish to communicate. It is anticipated that recipients can benefit from this information in ways that will cause their decision making to improve. As Derryberry (1952) has wisely explained, however, "The health educator should take into account the information and beliefs that people have about health and the causes of illness":

> All people, including primitive cultures, have their own theories about maintaining health and curing sickness. These theories may provide feelings of as much security for those who hold them as do the explanations based on modern science. The magical systems and traditions providing this security are found among people in all areas of the world. Most individuals use these magical systems to build their own concepts of life. For example, they may believe that taking three mouthfuls of water after cleaning their teeth, sleeping on one special side, taking deep breaths on rising, and many other rituals, will exercise a direct influence on their health.
>
> The health education worker who thinks that ignorant souls thirsting after knowledge will be glad to accept his views based on modern medical science is doomed to repeated failure. He underestimates the forces that maintain the processes underlying magic thinking about health. He will be unable to understand the anxieties that every individual experiences when his dearly fostered outlook on life and the world threatens to be shattered by the intrusion of other ideas (p. 3).

Health educators depend on other health professionals (including physicians, nurses, epidemiologists, and biostatisticians) to provide their knowledge of the theory and principles of a given problem or condition. In addition, health educators draw on resources such as voluntary health agencies, research, books, and government agencies to assemble their teaching materials.

Health educators are generalists who initially have little knowledge of the specific content of a problem, except in cases where they have gained knowledge through prior experience. Some health professionals have interpreted this generalism as a weakness: "Health educators don't know anything about a disease process because they have never been involved with its treatment." In fact, health educators' lack of a specific expertise provides for greater objectivity than is found in the more precise health disciplines, enhancing a needed understanding of the consumer's perspective on the problem.

For the health educator, the essential skill is the ability to ask the right questions, at the right time, to the right people. In other words, "How, and to whom, do we ask the questions in order to get the answers necessary to understand the nature of a given need?" To get these answers, health educators must ask, What is the need? Whom does it affect? What are the factors associated with its occurrence? What is the natural history of the condition? How does it affect persons over time? What actions can one take to prevent its occurrence? What actions can one take to lessen or alter its impact? Answers to these questions become the body of knowledge that forms the content of instruction.

Research and Evaluation

One of the important assumptions of health education practice is that a given educational intervention will effect a given outcome in a given setting. Health educators obviously need to know if change actually occurs and what critical factors are associated with the occurrence. Thus, a variety of research topics are of interest to the health educator. What is the distribution of learning opportunities within a setting? An environment? What are the major determinants of these learning opportunities? What are the critical components of the educational intervention? From an evaluative perspective, health educators will also ask, What methods produce a desired outcome? What are the impacts of these methods upon outcomes? Are there side effects associated with specific methods?

Health educators must be able to evaluate the products of their research at a variety of levels. All research materials associated with the specific problem must be evaluated for their relevance. The potential of each learning opportunity must be evaluated in relation to a desired outcome. (A more in-depth discussion of outcomes can be found in Chapter 8.)

Planning and Policy Formulation

By definition, health education programs are planned education interventions. By the word *planned,* we mean that they are structured according to a predetermined time and place, with written objectives, suggested methods, and a documented evaluation of the process. In the words of the APHA Policy Statement,

> Crucial to the success of an educational endeavor are the managerial elements common to all program planning. These are: Identification of problems, analysis of alternative approaches, setting objectives, assignment of resources, preparation of staff to carry out the function and monitoring performance. An organization base and sustained administrative and budgetary support are required.
>
> The focus of an educational program may be on individual and family practices. Different timetables, target audiences and methods may need to be selected depending on the problems and objectives. In developing the education program design, special attention must be given to involving members of the target population in the planning process and to determining their previous social, environmental and educational experiences (1978, p. 4).

A health educator must first determine the desired outcomes appropriate for a given setting within the boundaries set by the policymakers of the setting. This step, called the needs assessment, involves working with people to define needs and set goals. Next, the health educator must plan and develop programs that are consistent with the goals of the organization. This design step also involves working with people, principally policymakers, and includes both a review of alternative approaches to meeting needs and the establishment of priorities for needs and programs. Finally, for the educational intervention to occur, the health educator must address the following questions: In what facility will the learning opportunity occur? How will the content and process be organized? Who will pay the educators for their services? Who will provide the actual teaching? And, to whom will these educators be accountable for the content and the process of the instruction? A written description of the answers to these questions becomes the needs-objectives-methods-evaluation plan that formed a portion of our original formula for the potential of a learning opportunity (see Table 5.1, p. 97). Once the plan is implemented, the health educator can begin to evaluate it.

Organization and Administration

After a health education program is written, someone is assigned the responsibility of carrying it out. Largely, this responsibility involves organizing resources. Any planned and structured program characteristically has resources (facility, personnel, budget, and materials) that are used in the implementation of the program. A usual part of a health educator's task is to manage these resources in ways that will maximize the effectiveness and efficiency of the program.

From an organizational perspective, the health educator might write job descriptions, define procedures for accountability, establish schedules, and evaluate progress toward goals. From an administrative perspective, he or she may supervise personnel, prepare a budget, or submit quarterly expenditure reports. In addition, the health educator may evaluate and purchase a variety of teaching materials such as films, books, and pamphlets.

Coordination and Supervision

Coordination and supervision encompasses the whole activity of working with people. Health educators probably bring to their work more highly developed skills in group facilitation than any other member of the health team. These skills enable a health educator to be an effective coordinator of the entire health education process. In essence, health educators work with other people who, in turn, work with other people to provide a wide range of health education services. Inevitably this work requires a high degree of coordination.

For example, Lucy K. works as a patient educator at St. Mary's Hospital, where she has organized a program for diabetics. When a diabetic patient is admitted to the hospital, she is notified and then meets with the floor supervisor to develop a patient education plan. It will then be the floor supervisor's responsibility to see that the patient, during hospitalization, receives instruction regarding proper diet, use of insulin, and self-monitoring of blood-sugar levels. Periodically, Lucy checks back with the supervisor to answer questions and to provide additional materials. She will also review records on a monthly basis and assess the quality of the continuity of instruction.

The Program-Planning Process in Health Education

Several approaches can be used to describe how health educators engage in the practice of developing educational interventions. Most approaches are called models of health education program planning. The most widely known are Green's PRECEDE Framework for Health Education Planning, Sullivan's Comprehensive Health Education Model, and Ross and Mico's Model for Health Education Planning. Each model provides a slightly different perspective and warrants our review for the consideration of the diverse approaches to the process.

Three Planning Models for Health Education

Green's PRECEDE model (see Figure 7.1, pp. 130–31) shows seven phases that build on one another and lead to the identification of specific problems. In phases 1 and 2, Green focuses on identification of health problems as they relate to the "quality of life." In phase 3, he makes an important distinction between the bahavioral and nonbehavioral causes of a health problem; in phases 4 and 5, which he calls the educational diagnosis, he identifies the predisposing, enabling, and reinforcing factors that result in the behavioral causes identified in phase 3. Phase 6 involves the development of the health education components of a health program and its implementation. Finally, phase 7 (not pictured) identifies evaluation as an essential part of the total process.

Sullivan's Comprehensive Health Education Model (see Figure 7.2, pp. 132–33) lists six steps in health education planning, operation, and evaluation. The first is a classic statement on health education: it simply says, "Involve people." This step includes identifying the individuals affected, locating skilled personnel, and defining roles and relationships. The second step is goal setting, which is related to health status, health education practices, and resources. The third step, defining problems, is done by determining health service gaps that are linked to personal practices and to the lack of available resources. The fourth step is to design plans, which includes identifying and evaluating available programs and preparing written statements concerning objectives, activities, timetables, and resources. The fifth step, to conduct activities, involves obtaining funds, personnel, and facilities and developing policies and procedures necessary for implementing the plans. Finally, the sixth step is to evaluate results so that they either reinforce or substantiate the desired objectives and whether or not the objectives are being met.

Ross and Mico's Model for Health Education Planning is also designed in six phases and includes many of the same steps as Sullivan's model (see Table 7.1, pp. 134–35). An interesting feature of the model, first developed by Mico in 1966, is the delineation of a content, method, and process dimension for each phase.

Diagnostic Versus Needs-Assessment Approaches

Of the three models we have reviewed, Green's PRECEDE Framework has received the most acceptance because it has been tested in several different settings. Despite its use as a planning tool, however, we have found that some health educators fundamentally disagree with its perspective.

Green's perspective is based on the traditional public health approach. That is, by emphasizing the diagnosis of problems, he automatically assumes the exclusive, prescriptive approach of a "medical" model. Historically, public health has been defined as the diagnosis and treatment of the body politic. In this view, the public health official (or other public health professional) is seen as the physician, and the community is the patient. Public health disciplines, therefore, diagnose and treat a community much as a physician would diagnose and treat a patient.

Many health educators are uncomfortable with this prescriptive approach because it places public health professionals in an authoritarian position. By its very nature, the prescriptive approach presumes an authoritarian doctor-patient relationship. According to the theory of the distinguished sociologist Talcott Parsons on this relationship, "The patient (and usually his family) is by definition characterized by helplessness, lack of knowledge, and profound emotional involvement. As a result of this combination of factors, it is almost impossible to expect him or his family to exercise rational judgment with respect to his illness or treatment. He must, therefore, have complete confidence in his doctor and accept his judgment unquestioningly on authority" (quoted by Somers, 1977, p. 6).

One of the unfortunate ramifications of this authoritarian mode, Somers (1977) explains, is "the concept of the un-cooperative patient," which has "become deeply embedded in medical mores." Somers continues: "A recent study in the outpatient clinic of a teaching hospital, for example, found that students, faculty, and other medical personnel readily agreed on the definition: a patient is un-cooperative when he is stubborn, when he won't recognize that help is being given to him, when he refuses

Figure 7.1 *Green's* PRECEDE *Framework for Health Education Planning*

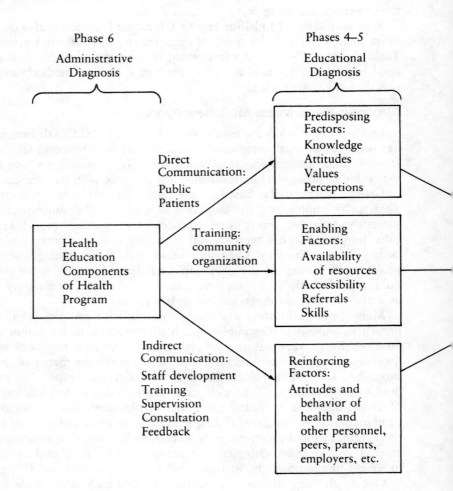

Source: L. W. Green *et al.*, "Health Education Today and the PRECEDE Framework," in *Health Education Planning: A Diagnostic Approach* (Palo Alto, Calif.: Mayfield Publishing Company, 1980), pp. 14–15.

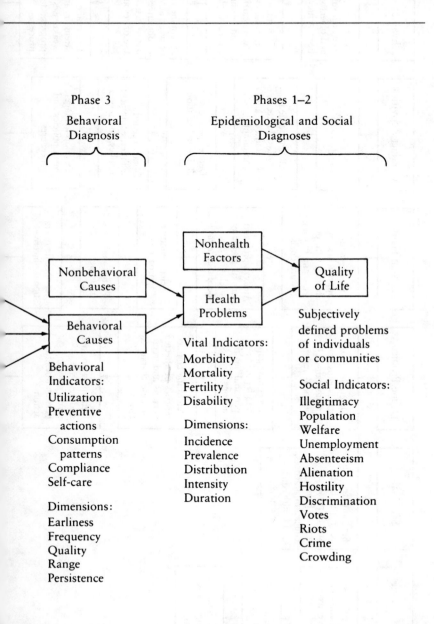

Phase 3
Behavioral
Diagnosis

Phases 1–2
Epidemiological and Social
Diagnoses

Nonhealth
Factors

Nonbehavioral
Causes

Quality
of Life

Behavioral
Causes

Health
Problems

Subjectively
defined problems
of individuals
or communities

Behavioral
Indicators:
Utilization
Preventive
  actions
Consumption
  patterns
Compliance
Self-care

Vital Indicators:
Morbidity
Mortality
Fertility
Disability

Social Indicators:
Illegitimacy
Population
Welfare
Unemployment
Absenteeism
Alienation
Hostility
Discrimination
Votes
Riots
Crime
Crowding

Dimensions:
Earliness
Frequency
Quality
Range
Persistence

Dimensions:
Incidence
Prevalence
Distribution
Intensity
Duration

Figure 7.2 *Sullivan's Comprehensive Health Education Model*

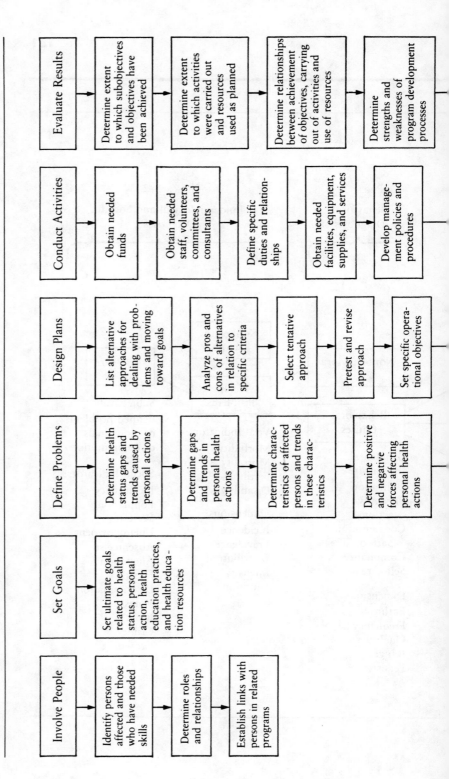

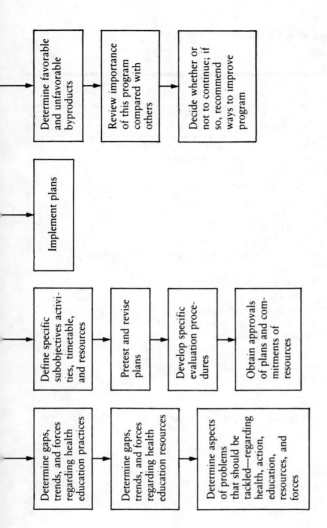

Source: Adapted from D. Sullivan, "Model for Comprehensive, Systematic Program Development in Health Education," *Health Education Report* 1, no. 1 (November–December 1973): 4–5.

Table 7.1 *Ross and Mico's Model for Health Education Planning*

	Content Dimension
Phase 6 Evaluation	4. Knowledge of problem and client system 3. Technology of feedback systems 2. Language and systems 1. Nature of evaluation
Phase 5 Implementation	4. Writing skills 3. Dynamics of problem solving 2. Knowledge of subject and content T&TA being provided for 1. Knowledge of plan, how it is to work
Phase 4 Planning/ Programming	3. Nature of political process 2. Systems analysis and management science 1. Techniques of planning
Phase 3 Goal setting	5. Theory of change 4. MBO technology 3. Forecasting 2. Nature of policy 1. Role of goals, how to set them, measure
Phase 2 Needs Assessment	4. Relevance of data 3. Language and systems 2. Data sources 1. Standards and criteria
Phase 1 Initiate	3. Power and influence structures, community organization, culture 2. Contract terminology and resources 1. Knowledge of problem and client system

Source: H. S. Ross and P. R. Mico, *Theory and Practice in Health Education* (Palo Alto, Calif.: Mayfield Publishing Company, 1980), pp. 214–15. First developed by Paul Mico in 1966, this model has been updated periodically as continuing application and experience have made further refinements possible.

Method Dimension	Process Dimension
4. Redefine problem and standards	4. Consensus of new definitions
3. Feedback to activity, reporting, accountability	3. Communication, threat reduction
2. Data collection and analysis	2. Learning, assimilation
1. Clarify evaluation measures	1. Agreement
4. Reporting	4. Communications
3. Problem solving	3. Creativity, conflict resolution, win-win
2. Training and technical assistance, consultation	2. Skill development, helping
1. Initiate activity	1. Communications, orientations
3. Negotiate commitments, MOA's	3. Negotiation
2. Design management systems and tools	2. Role clarification, communications
1. Develop implementation plan	1. Understanding and commitment
5. Determine strategies for implementation	5. Consensus
4. Select goals and objectives	4. Decision making, consenus
3. Alternative goals statement, force-field analysis	3. Reality testing, creative problem solving
2. Link to policy development	2. Understanding of process and roles
1. Establish criteria for goals	1. Agreement
4. Describe nature and extent of problem	4. Reduce fantasy by fact
3. Data collection and analysis	3. Open communications, sensitivity to data sources
2. Determine data to be collected	2. Agreement
1. Identify and review present criteria	1. Agreement on starting point
3. Organize concerned parties	3. Involvement, leadership, values clarification
2. Develop initial contract	2. Legitimacy, commitment, trust, readiness
1. Entry or intervention strategy, force-field analysis, interviewing	1. Unfreezing, threat reduction, credibility, awareness of need

to accept his condition or when he fails to appreciate the efforts that have been expended on his behalf" (p. 67).

Many thoughtful health educators have disagreed with this traditional public health view of an authoritarian, elitist relationship with their community, whether they be patients or target groups. Instead, these health educators have maintained a democratic point of view that seeks to understand people within the context of their culture and give full credit to people's knowledge, beliefs, and practices. Because they believe in involving people and making them an integral part of the decision-making processes that affect their own lives and the community at large, these health educators use a "theory and principles" intervention strategy, rather than a "prescriptive" strategy. They assume that people, with complete disclosure of information and an understanding of consequences, are free to decide for themselves.

Another facet of the role of health educator as a teacher's teacher is becoming evident in the medical profession, as doctors are beginning to be acknowledged as educators. As Somers (1977) notes,

> "Educational" may suggest the essence of the newly emerging relationship of doctor and patient just as the "traditional" relationship is frequently identified as "authoritarian." The terms are not mutually exclusive; the overlap is also evident in the types of relationship they suggest. Yet the differences are fundamental. Where the authoritarian relationship assumes—and does not discourage—the continued dependence of the patient on the doctor's superior knowledge and wisdom, the educational relationship aims to help the patient understand his illness or problem, to assume maximum responsibility for his own recovery, and to overcome his dependence.
>
> Where the old relationship was one of unbridgeable inequality, the new is essentially democratic, although never quite reaching the point of equality. The doctor remains in full charge of the diagnosis and treatment, but makes of his patient an informed, active participant, with full knowledge of facts and the probable consequences of alternative courses of action. The relationship is basically secular, although it cannot fully dispel the elements of mysticism and faith that overhang the continuing uncertainties and fears surrounding life-and-death situations (p. 67).

Rather than focusing on problems, and in fact labeling people themselves as "problems" and therefore viewing them as victims, health educators have maintained the perspective that people have needs. *Problem,* in this sense, is synonomous with something undesirable that must be dealt with by society. *Needs,* on the other hand, are conditions that people desire—in this case, improved health. Although this distinction may appear to be a matter of semantics, few health educators have practiced under the auspices of a diagnostic approach. They have always used the term *needs assessment* to describe the process of involving people in determining what needs to be changed (i.e., the identification of needs) and what actions to take.

The Health Educator as Program Planner

All the models we have discussed include a step that has to do with "implementing" a program. However, they do not specify in detail how this implementation occurs, in spite of the fact that it is the most important step in a health education program. Thus, we need to go beyond these models to consider the planning process in greater detail.

The planning process has been traditionally characterized as an "abstract model of perfect rationality in social decision-making" (Freedman, 1967). The underlying notion is that the process of planning enhances rationality because of the intellectual stages one goes through in logical problem solving. This concept of rational problem solving characterizes all approaches to planning health services. The process begins with a method of identifying problems, then proceeds through analysis of the problem, identification and specification of alternative solutions, selection of alternatives for implementation, and evaluation.

Logical problem solving has two major characteristics: the gathering of information and the application of measures to test, explain, and control events (i.e., to create planned change). The assumptions on which the process is based are (1) that factual knowledge is a prerequisite to adequate decision making, (2) that this knowledge can be used to solve problems, and (3) that this knowledge is attainable through the use of inductive and deductive reasoning. Thus, planners not only draw conclusions, but test these ideas by applying them to the world at large to determine their validity. Their reasoning is based on selected information collected on related events in order to make reliable predictions of events yet unknown. In effect, planners are obligated to test the social theories upon which plans are based if they are to explain, and ultimately control, events.

How does the health educator, as a planner, solve problems through the use of information? As Biller (1969) suggests, this process is analogous to the classic scientific procedure of the null hypothesis. There is much similarity between translating the grand designs of planners into concrete actions and validating scientific theory through basic research. Both processes are based on rational thinking, which uses knowledge as a common denominator for making decisions about the future. The processes of inductive and deductive reasoning are the same. In a similar vein, both scientific propositions and plans can be proved fallacious by comparing them with the world of reality. The scientist moves constantly between hypothesis and data, seeking to construct a model that is consistent with the pattern observed. Similarly, the planner tests plans through implementation to determine their effectiveness in establishing rational control over social processes. Biller (1969) refers to this as a "development process," synonomous with "learning." He equates "learning" with the procedure of the null hypothesis. The planner goes through a process of testing out the specific conditions under which a hypothesis or plan does not apply. The essential difference between the planner and the scientist is that whereas the researcher pursues knowledge for its own worth, the planner seeks knowledge to guide actions. Knowledge improves interventions, which create changes that otherwise would not occur.

Given this perspective on the planning process, the evaluation of health education programs becomes much more significant. It is the sole instrument which the health educator can use to validate plans and the health education theories on which they are based. Thus, evaluation is fundamentally important because it tests whether a planned intervention succeeds or fails by testing the underlying assumptions on which the educational intervention operates.

This view of the planning process has several implications for the role of the health educator in health education practice. First, it emphasizes that the health educators, like scientists, develop plans (needs-objectives-methods-evaluation statements that are hypotheses) and are obligated to test them (through implementation) in the world at large in order to validate their value, appropriateness, efficiency, and effectiveness. Consequently, to define the health education planning process as "the creation of an educational intervention" inadequately describes the planning process or the role of the health educator as a planner.

Second, health educators should give particular attention to the evaluation of programs because it is the single technique that introduces greater rationality into policymaking. Health educators are, in effect, "learning by doing," and evaluation is the mechanism for processing and retaining the experiences from which they have learned.

Third, health educators should not be disillusioned by the failure of programs. Unsuccessful planning is fundamentally more important than successful planning. According to Peterson (1968), "the true test of a plan is its failure, which is parallel to the negation of the scientific theory." The health educator should recognize that the identification of deficiencies in a plan is the principal way in which the science of health education, as a whole, progresses. Just as scientists are spurred on by the failure of experiments to explain phenomena, so are health educators stimulated to arrive at alternative plans that more effectively produce the desired change. Health educators are obligated to carefully examine unsuccessful plans to determine the reasons for their failure. As with scientists, the ultimate test of the skills of health educators is to explain why a phenomenon happened. Health educators must identify and differentiate the reasons why their programs failed.

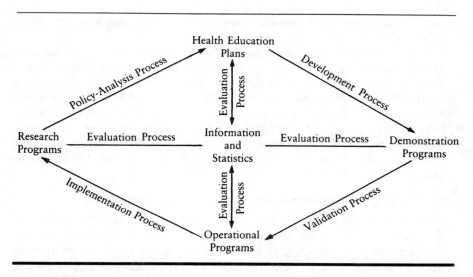

Figure 7.3 *A Conceptual Model for the Analysis of Health Education Planning and Resource Development*

A Model for Health Education Planning and Resource Development

At this point we would like to introduce our own concept of the health education planning process. Our proposed model, shown in Figure 7.3, establishes the minimum conceptual framework necessary for a scientifically disciplined study of the relationship between plan and implementation. A distinguishing feature of the model is that it separates process from end results. Each of the five major points in the model—health education plans, demonstration programs, operational programs, research programs, information and statistics—represents an end result of the planning process. The arrows that link these end results illustrate the process itself—the movement or sequence of events that occurs in health education program planning.

The Policy-Analysis Process and Health Education Plan

In our model, *policy analysis* means the process of needs assessment. In other words, the health education program plan (the statement of needs, objectives, methods, and evaluation) is an end result, or product, of a process of policy analysis, or needs assessment. Because the creation of a plan calls for the identification of needs and the analysis of alternative policies that could meet those needs, health educators draw on information and statistics derived from previous research, demonstrations, and operational programs. After appropriate analysis of this data, policy options are prepared and reviewed. If possible, projections of the costs and benefits of each option are calculated.

This process of policy analysis is largely based on inductive reasoning. Health educators attempt to resolve conflicting or overlapping goals through some system of rational choice. The end result of the process is a health education plan that is based on the best available knowledge about how a need can be met. This written document consists of specific objectives, as well as sets of strategies and substrategies, necessary to accomplish the objectives. To prepare such a plan, health educators begin by asking people, What needs to be changed? and, further, What can be changed within the context of a given setting?

The Development Process and Demonstration of Programs

Up to this point, our model has not departed from the way traditional theorists describe health education planning. The essential difference is that we will go a step further by linking the health education plan to its implementation. Our model does this by treating plans as hypotheses to be tested—hypotheses that require validation to demonstrate their effectiveness. Thus, health educators are obligated to follow their plan through a series of steps to test its worth and usefulness. The process of development involves the designation and funding of specific demonstration programs according to the overall requirements stated in the plan. Because planning is a deductive process, the design should be completed first. Then, depending on the significance of the need and the availability of resources, one or more demonstration programs should be established.

Health education demonstration programs test whether a set of services can operate within the context of a sociocultural, political, economic environment, and in a given setting, prior to the implementation of similar programs on a large-scale basis. The assumptions underlying health demonstration programs are (1) that investment of moneys can expand the capacity of the setting by establishing new health education services (i.e., new learning opportunities are present and available), (2) that these new services can be established on a permanent basis (i.e., the services must survive after the initial demonstration period), (3) that these educational services have an impact on the health status of the target population, and (4) that knowledge of the costs and resources of the program can be used to estimate requirements for operational programs.

The Validation Process and Operational Programs

The validation process concerns assessing the results of one or more demonstration programs, first, to contribute to the development of theory about the programs' impact and survival within particular settings and, second, to provide a basis for generalizations about programs that can be used as models for possible replication and expansion. Validation involves reviewing evaluations of separate demonstration programs to validate the program assumptions upon which the demonstrations operate. For those demonstrations that fail, an attempt is made to differentiate between failure of the program and failure of the validity assumptions. Successful demonstrations are examined to determine why and under what conditions they were successful. After this validation process, an implementation plan is prepared that reflects the experiences learned during the demonstration. In this manner, major unknown variables can be determined prior to implementation on a large-scale basis, and more precise estimates can be made regarding the resources required. Thus, the products of the validation process are operational programs based on a sound rationale of research, planning, and demonstrations.

The Implementation Process and Research Programs

Once an implementation plan is prepared, the program itself may be quite similar to a demonstration program, except that implementation is on a much larger scale. The planners hope that all major mistakes identified during the evaluation of the demonstration programs will have been avoided.

The major concern regarding the operation of programs is how to maintain a high level of efficiency while providing the health education services. Health education research enters the process at this point, because questions about access, quality, continuity, and efficiency are frequently raised that, to some degree, can be answered quantitatively. In effect, the problems of the implementation process form research questions for health education researchers. With appropriate designs and experimentation, researchers formulate possible answers to these questions, using information that becomes valuable data for future policy analysis and planning. In this manner, the health education planning cycle begins anew, and proceeds in an evolutionary pattern toward the provision of increasingly better organized and effective health education services.

The Evaluation Process and Information and Statistics

Our model is now almost complete except for the important function of evaluation and the assembling of information. We view evaluation as a process that produces information and statistics which can then be used to improve decision making. A major difference between our model and others is the role of evaluation. Instead of following implementation in the same manner in which the three previous models would place it, evaluation is viewed as an integral part of each phase. Thus, each arrow flowing toward the center of the model indicates a point at which plans, demonstrations, operational programs, and research programs are evaluated. Evaluation has the key function of testing and validating program assumptions throughout the entire process.

Basic to a meaningful understanding of health education planning is the information-seeking behavior of the health educator, who must be able to assimilate large quantities of data from multiple sources. By placing the information-and-statistics end result in the center of the model, with arrows flowing both inward and outward, we have tried to illustrate the important function of information. Research, operational programs, and demonstration programs are important sources of data that flow into the information pool. This body of assembled data then serves as an intelligence center where evaluation findings are stored and specific findings are processed to become forecasts that help to improve future program plans.

Success and Failure in Health Education Practice

To illustrate the importance of the evaluation process as a major modality of learning about health education program practice, we need to review several types of errors that may result in program failure. For example, health educators have been accused of failing to integrate a substantial body of theory into actual practice. Critics cite an inability to bridge the gap between information provided to individuals and the individuals' resulting behavior, or an inability to deal with the overwhelming social forces that underlie the problem health educators face.

We rebut the criticism of health educators' inability to integrate theory into practice. Instead, we attribute the failures of health education practice, first, to an inability on the part of health educators to be able to understand the relationship between a given setting and the environment in which it must function and, second, to a lack of the skills necessary to create the specific outcomes required by a setting.

Types of Errors in Health Education Practice

Failures within health education practice generally fall into three categories. Looking again at the formula for the potential of a learning opportunity that we first stated in Table 5.1,

$$LO_p = (f) \, S + T + Ed \, (N{:}O{:}M{:}E) + Ln$$

we note that each variable may be the focus of an error that could result in practice failure.

One obvious source of error in an educational intervention has to do with the dose-response relationship. (By "dose," we mean the amount and type of intervention required to produce a specific outcome.) An error of this nature is characterized by an inappropriate method or objective that operates on too much or too little information. In effect, the "dose" has not been appropriately matched with the need.

For example, if a six-year-old child asks its mother, "Where did I come from?" and the mother replies, "From Paducah, Kentucky," a potential learning opportunity has been completely missed. In fact, the child was asking for some basic information about childbirth. Playing the scene out another way, the mother might have gone into elaborate details of the fertilization process and looked up to see that her child had fallen asleep. Because her long and involved explanation gave too much information for a small child to absorb, she again would miss a learning opportunity because of an inappropriate method.

A second type of error, which occurs frequently, involves a miscue or confused signal that results in a lack of appropriate timing. Recognizing when a learning opportunity has great potential is crucial to successful educational interventions. Such knowledge comes with experience or through the continued evaluation of programs. For example, it is known that women are very receptive to birth-control information during the first six weeks after the delivery of their baby. If an intervention occurs during this time, the mother is much more likely to accept a birth-control method than if the same intervention was made available to her six months postpartum.

A third type of error—perhaps the most serious for the health education practitioner—involves a misidentification of the specific needs of the learner around which the intervention is being designed. Although the result has sometimes been interpreted as a failure of theory, it is, in fact, a program failure. To misidentify the needs of the learner suggests that the health educator does not have a working knowledge of his or her target population. Perhaps the health educator has not involved appropriate people. Whatever its source, erronous information means that objectives and methods are doomed to fail. And the implications of a program failure unfortunately spill over into other areas of health education practice.

By misidentification of needs, the health educator may not only fail to positively affect health status but, in fact, may exacerbate the whole condition. For example, in a study of lead poisoning among children in certain black neighborhoods in Cleveland, Ohio, researchers mistakenly focused on the need to change the behavior of mothers. By claiming that Southern black mothers were permissive—allowing their children's oral behavior to include eating lead paint—they shifted the blame and responsibility to the mothers and away from both the poor housing conditions in which the mothers and children lived and the society that continued to allow these conditions to exist.

Variations In Skills and Settings

In this chapter, we have seen clearly that health education practice must vary among settings. Although the same combination of skills is necessary to practice health education everywhere, the way in which these skills are combined will often differ according to the setting. Figure 7.4

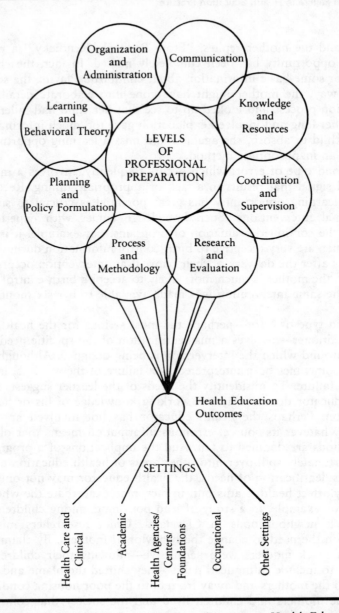

Figure 7.4   *The Interaction of Skills and Settings in Health Education Practice*

Source: This model was originally developed by Elena Sliepcevich, Alan Henderson, and Ira J. Bates.

contrasts skills and settings and illustrates some of these combinations. For example, the skill of program planning and policy formulation in a school setting is referred to as *curriculum design;* in a clinical setting, it is known as a *patient education program planning.* In each instance, the health educator needs to know the language that is specific to that setting and be familiar with the procedures of the setting in order to be able successfully to apply the program-planning process. In another example, learning and behavioral theory in a school setting is applied to the individual and the classroom; in a health agency setting, it may be applied to the individual, but is more frequently applied to a segment of the population or the whole community.

Another variation, in process and methodology, can be seen by contrasting school and health agencies. In schools the setting is structured in such a way that discrete times for units of instruction are provided. In health agencies, however, since there is no specific place where a unit of instruction can occur, it is difficult to provide a specific timeframe. Consequently, health educators in health agencies must integrate their educational programs into the provision of other services or provide them in settings designed specifically for instruction.

Variation is also found in the skill area of research and evaluation. In the school setting, evaluation is referred to as *testing and measurement,* whereas in the clinical setting, it is called the *documentation of results.* The school setting is largely concerned with measuring individual performance; the health agency setting is more concerned with measuring behavior change in the population.

These are just a few examples of the variations of terms and of levels of skills required to practice health education. Knowing that these variations exist and being able to appropriately apply specific skills in a given setting is the difference between a good health educator with a successful practice and one who will meet with little success.

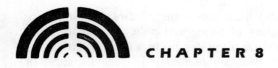

CHAPTER 8

Outcomes and Evaluation in Health Education

In Chapter 4, which was devoted to the development of an evolving theory of change, we described four types of change: first-order changes from one way of behaving to another for (1) individuals and (2) organizations or societies, and second-order changes in ways of behaving, also for (3) individuals and (4) organizations or societies. We further defined micro change, as change in a small unit—a person—and macro change as change in a large unit—an organization, community, or society. We have also previously stated that the process of change is effected by the action of a planned intervention. We will now more fully define the result of this change, the outcome, as the result of a planned intervention that aims at a change in a unit (characterized as an individual, organization, community, or society) and that will have a positive effect on the health status of the person or persons that constitute that unit.

Figure 8.1 shows us all the possible combinations of outcomes that can result from change inverventions. First, there are the four outcomes we have already mentioned: change from one way of behaving to another and change in ways of behaving, for both a person and an organization. Additional combinations are (1) organizational change from one behavior to another that leads to individual change from one behavior to another; (2) individual change in ways of behaving that leads to organizational change from one behavior to another; (3) organizational change from one behavior to another that leads to individual change in ways of behaving; and (4) organizational change in ways of behaving that leads to any or all of the following: individual change from one behavior to another, individual

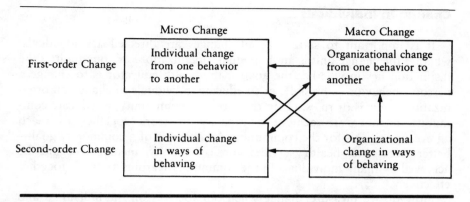

Figure 8.1   *The Interaction of Types and Levels of Change*

change in ways of behaving, and organizational change from one behavior to another.

In our case study in Chapter 4 concerning carpal tunnel syndrome (CTS), for example, the employer's redesign of the sewing machine should lead to workers' behavior that reduces their risk of CTS (the first combination noted above). We illustrated the second combination by the example of an intervention that facilitates the development of self-reliance in the workers, which in turn would lead the employer (organization) to replace the piecework pay system with a work-week salary structure. The third combination would result if the employer's redesign of the machine, to alleviate hand motions leading to CTS, would then lead to workers' awareness that they have been placed at risk of injury by the piecework method. Workers might then change their attitudes about this method of production and payment and either ask to be retrained for a new job in the shop or resign.

A change by the employer (organizational change) from the piecework pay system to a work-week salary would exemplify the fourth combination we noted above. Such a change would eliminate worker behavior that can result in CTS. It could lead to a further change in the workers' consciousness (the piecework method is injurious), to a change in attitude by workers, and therefore to a change in their behavior relevant to piecework. This change could also lead workers to ask for other changes in organizational behavior, such as worker input into setting salary schedules. It should be clear from our illustration of combination four that a second-order macro-change intervention can influence behavior on the other three change levels. Second-order macro change, therefore, is the most powerful change intervention in the possession of a change agent.

Change in Individuals

It is important to state that all changes are directed at individuals, whether the change unit is an individual, organization, or community. The distinction lies in whether the goal of the health educator is to change a person's behavior or lifestyle, or to educate individuals to change an organization's norms or rules, or, in the case of a community, to educate community members to achieve a capacity to work together to reach agreed-upon goals for the community. An example of a community goal—better access to health services for community members—could be achieved by many individuals in the community learning to work together effectively.

How do we measure change when our focus is on the individual and our goal is either change from one form of behavior to another or lifestyle change? The most direct measure of outcome is the attainment of the desired goal; that is, has the target individual changed his or her behavior in the desired direction? Has, for example, Mr. Jones stopped smoking? Has Mrs. Jones changed her diet? Changes in an individual that can lead to action supporting or inhibiting health behavior can also be measured by noting changes in the person's knowledge, attitudes, beliefs, and values.

Green, Kreuter, Deeds, and Partridge (1980) refer to knowledge, beliefs, values, and attitudes as predisposing factors that relate "to the motivation of an individual or group to act" (p. 70). They believe that those factors may either support or inhibit health behavior. Knowledge represents the amount of information an individual has about a health practice. This includes information about the consequences to the individual of poor health behavior, what the appropriate health behaviors are, and how they reduce the individual's risk of becoming sick. The other factors—beliefs, values, and attitudes—represent the personal preferences that an individual or group brings to an educational experience.

A belief is a conviction that an object or situation is true. Faith, trust, and value express belief statements. Green et al. (1980) cite the following examples as health-related belief statements: "I don't believe that medication can work. If this diet won't work for him, it sure isn't going to work for me" (p. 72). The Health Belief Model developed by Becker and Maiman (1974) attempts to predict health-related behavior change in terms of certain belief patterns. The sequence of belief events that must occur if behavior is to change is as follows:

1. The person must believe that his or her health is in jeopardy.
2. The person must perceive the potential seriousness of the condition in terms of pain or discomfort, time lost from work, economic difficulties, and so forth.
3. On assessing the circumstances, the person must believe that bene-

fits stemming from the healthy behavior outweigh the costs and are indeed possible and within his or her grasp.

4. There must be a "cue to action" or a precipitating force that makes the person feel the need to take action.

A value is a guide to a wide range of behaviors. We may place a value on either a mode of conduct or the result of conduct. Good health is generally considered an end result that health-related behaviors are directed to achieve. It is also possible, of course, for us to place a personal value on modes of conduct that are in conflict with an end result we also value. For example, an individual may value good health, but may also value cigarette smoking or excessive consumption of alcohol. The resolution of a value conflict or the clarification of that individual's values is an important change that must precede a change in behavior.

Our final predisposing factor, attitude, is subject to many definitions in the literature of behavioral sciences. The two key concepts that define attitudes are, first, that an attitude is a constant feeling and is always directed toward an object (toward a person, action, or an idea) and, second, that an attitude is always evaluative (the object can be assessed as good or bad). There is a strong belief among social scientists, based on a long history of research, that if you change attitudes, behavior change will follow.

Although goal attainment does represent a direct measure of behavior change, measurements of change in knowledge, beliefs, values, and attitudes can be indirect measures of behavior change. An increase in knowledge may not alone lead directly to behavior change. Nevertheless, Cartwright (1949), Farquhar (1977), and others have found evidence of a meaningful association between an increase in knowledge and a desired behavior change. For example, school health education has long justified its existence according to the rationale that information delivered to students produces knowledge, which leads to actions that result in a healthier life.

In our discussion of interventions we remarked that prescriptive interventions (those providing information, using confrontation, and giving directive advice) lead to individuals changing from one behavior to another. This kind of change generally reflects a gain in knowledge or a modification of a belief. Changes in ways of behaving, on the other hand, tend to reflect changes in the attitudes or values held by individuals.

If, for example, a mother complains that she has trouble putting her year-old infant to sleep, she might be directed to put the infant to bed and to allow him to cry for 30 minutes. She would be specifically directed not to interfere and would be told that she must not impose her wish to be with the infant or to interfere with his need to sleep. This combined use of direction and information could succeed in changing her belief about her infant's need for her attendance on him at bedtime. An alternative approach to this problem would be to explore with the mother her need to be with her infant at this time. Mother herself may reveal her own fears about falling asleep. She may have attributed these fears to her infant and believe that he must share them. These fears in mother can have their origins in her negative attitude toward losing consciousness. Once the infant's mother understands this attitude and can perceive that she is transferring it onto her child, she realizes that this is her unconscious fear and is part of her lifestyle. She can now change her attitude toward herself and, as a result of this change in a way of behaving, also change her behavior toward her child.

Change in Organizations

How do we measure change in institutions or organizations? Organizational change means that the norms and the values of an organization have been modified in more or less permanent ways so that certain identified problems are unlikely to interfere with organizational effectiveness or with the satisfaction of the group members. For example, conflicts could be handled directly rather than avoided, organizational goals might be clarified, and a majority of the organization's members would evidence a reasonable committment to these goals. There would be confidence that the leadership is ready to provide strong and continued guidance, and the group members would be acquiring the skills to implement the new norms and values in their work.

An immediate measure of the effectiveness of change is to determine whether these desired goals have been attained. These changes may be approached through the use of prescriptive or group-dynamic methods of intervention. Suppose, for example, you are asked to develop a program to reduce the number of work hours lost due to alcoholism among employees. You might try a two-pronged approach, first, providing greater information to workers about the negative effects of alcohol and, second, asking employees who have a "drinking problem" to meet with a foreman who has been instructed to confront workers with job-performance problems that are believed to be the result of their drinking. The ultimate goal of the intervention is to increase worker productivity; the intermediate goals are a reduction in alcoholism and an improvement in health status among plant employees. This approach would seek to ameliorate an organizational problem by changing problem drinking behavior among employees. An alternative approach would be, first, to develop a diagnosis of what organizational norms and values are in conflict with employee effectiveness and satisfaction and, second, to develop a program to change or modify those norms and values. This approach is based on the assumption that employees are stressed by organizational conflicts and that alcoholism is, in many individuals, a means of coping with excess stress. Following this change strategy, you might conduct an experimental workshop with small groups, with the goal of changing worker and management attitudes and values within the context of organizational norms and values. These may include conflict management, performance approach, and communication skills.

Lewin's (1948) now classic analysis of the process of planned change is the model for this alternative approach to change. As you recall, he identified the first step in this process as "unfreezing." By unfreezing he meant identifying the need to give up habitual or stereotyped behaviors that are well integrated into an individual's behavior. All of the interventions (discussed in the previous chapter) that permit the client system to understand its present level of functioning, and the negative consequences of this functioning, can be seen as unfreezing procedures. Unfreezing would also include encouraging the client to consider behavioral alternatives or new norms.

In Lewin's second step in planned change, "moving to a new level," new behaviors are attempted, and the client system develops some skills in these behaviors. At this point, the intervenor may need to assist the client with encouragement. Since any new set of behaviors is initially awkward and uncomfortable, the tendency to give them up and return to an older and more comfortable mode of operation is a typical and understandable response. As we suggested earlier, the intervenor's level of activity during this phase is intensive, as he or she organizes and manages team-building workshops, skills-development programs, and other strategies to integrate the new behaviors.

The final stage of Lewin's approach to planned change is "freezing" the group's behavior at the new level. By freezing (actually "refreezing"), Lewin meant the stabilization and generalization of change. In other words, the new behaviors have become part of the client's normal behavior and are self-sustaining. In the terms of our earlier discussion, the changes that the client and the intervenor have collaboratively agreed upon have been institutionalized.

In the first type of drinking-behavior program we outlined, outcome measures can be based on gains in information and changes in beliefs among the employees as well as on measurable changes in behavior. Outcome measures in the second, Lewin-based approach can be gauged by changes within the organization. We have selected some examples from the literature on organizational change as illustrations of the kind of outcome measures currently in use. Greiner (1967), for example, compared 18 different interventions and found that successful ones shared three characteristics: (1) strong internal and external pressures for organizational change, (2) a gradual involvement of many levels of the organization (including top management) in the process of change, and (3) more shared decision making instead of unrelated or delegated decisions.

In a comparison of 67 published reports of organizational change efforts, Dunn and Swierczek (1977) found support for 3 of 11 major hypotheses about planned change. The interventions were more successful (1) if the client and the intervenor had a collaborative relationship, (2) if the intervenor adopted a participative orientation rather than that of an expert, and (3) if the intervention strategy involved high levels of participation in the change effort by the client system. Among the 8 remaining hypotheses that received weak or no support were those concerning differences between profit-making and nonprofit organizations, stable and unstable task environments, internal and external intervenors, single versus multiple-level interventions, and total versus partial organizational involvement. Dunn and Swierczek's data analysis offers strong support for the collaborative, participative approach.

Similar support is found in the work of Glaser (1977), who compared the impact of four different intervenors on four residential treatment centers for disturbed children. His detailed analysis of these intervenors led him to conclude that effective interventions must be open to input from the entire client system and must maintain flexibility about the intervention. The intervenor's role needs to be carefully defined. Moreover, his or her role as an agent facilitating two-way communication with the client system needs to be strongly supported by influential persons in that system, ideally the top management of the organization and their immediate staff.

Change In Communities

We can also examine models of community change in terms of first- and second-order change. Here the problem of outcome depends in large part on the selection of the goals to be attained. Rothman (1968) has identified two major categories of goals discussed in the community organization literature: "task" and "process" goals.

> Task goals entail the completion of a concrete task or the solution of a delimited problem pertaining to the functioning of a community social system—delivery of services, establishment of new services, passing of specific social legislation. Process goals, or maintenance goals, are more oriented to system maintenance and capacity, with aims such as establishing cooperative working relationships among groups in the community, creating self-maintaining community problem solving structures, improving the power base of the community, stimulating wide interest and participation in community affairs, fostering collaborative attitudes and practices, and increasing indigenous leadership (p. 37).

Murray Ross (1955) characterizes this second set of goals as "community integration" and "community capacity." Process goals are concerned with a generalized or gross capacity of the community system to function over time; task goals, with the solution of delimited functional problems of the system.

In locality development, process goals are heavily emphasized. The community's capacity to become functionally integrated, engage in cooperative problem solving on a self-help basis, and utilize democratic processes is of central importance. Community practice in adult education makes citizen education the cardinal aim. Applied "group dynamics" professionals likewise assert the priority of "methodological" goals over "substantive" goals, viewed in terms of personal or community growth. The same orientation is found in theoretical writings in the field of community development, where improving the community's "mental health" is sometimes viewed as primary.

In the social-planning approach, stress is placed on task goals oriented toward the solution of substantive social problems. Social-planning organizations are often mandated specifically to deal with concrete social problems. Their official names signify this: mental health departments, city planning and urban renewal authorities, commissions on physical rehabilitation or alcoholism, and so on.

The social-action approach may lean in the direction of either task goals or process goals. Some social-action organizations, such as civil rights groups and cause-oriented organizations (welfare rights, trade unions), emphasize obtaining specific legislative outcomes (higher welfare allotments) or changing specific social practices (the hiring of more minorities by corporations). Usually these objectives entail the modification of policies of formal organizations. Other social-action groups lean more toward process goals, such as building a constituency with the ability to acquire and exercise power (as exemplified by Saul Alinsky and the Industrial Areas Foundation or the militant black power movement). This objective of building local-based power and decision-making centers transcends the solution of any given problem situation. Goals are often viewed as the result of changing the system rather than tinkering with small-scale or short-range problem situations. These small-scale activities are often pursued, however, because they are feasible and they help to build an organization. Creating power may be also associated with building personal self-esteem.

The locality-development, social-planning, and social-action approaches also tend to stress different change strategies. In locality development, strategies of consensus are stressed. These generally include discussion and communication among a wide range of different individuals, groups, and factors. In the social-planning model, fact finding about problems and the presentation of information are important strategies used to influence decision makers. In social action, strategies involving confrontation and direct action are emphasized as a means of creating change. Although there can be some overlapping of strategies in each model, it is clear that locality development emphasizes attitude and value change and that the two other approaches rely more heavily on information, confrontation, and direct action. To measure outcomes, therefore, we should look, in addition to goal attainment, primarily at changes in knowledge and beliefs in the social-action and social-planning approaches and at changes in attitudes and values in the locality-development approach.

Evaluation of Outcomes

All educational interventions aimed at changing health-related behavior are planned interventions. A health educator's first step in developing a program is to write a program plan. In Chapter 7, which focuses on the methods of health education, we have fully discussed the components of the program plan, which include concern for the client, purpose, objectives, methods of procedure, and evaluation. Now we will look at evaluation, the final stage of the program plan, as a way of measuring the outcomes of a program and its value to the clients. We begin with Weiss's (1972) excellent definition of evaluation as a way "to measure the effects of a program against the goals it set out to accomplish, as a means of contributing to subsequent decision making about the program and improving future programming" (p. 5). This definition includes the four major aspects of the evaluation process: (1) determining social purpose, (2) determining outcomes, (3) developing measurement criteria, and (4) selecting appropriate research methodology.

Social Purposes of Evaluations

Determining the social purpose of an evaluation is the most significant step in the evaluation process, since it establishes rules for the entire evaluation. In the process of appraisal, it is important to consider both who is conducting the evaluation, and for what purpose.

An evaluation is based on the value system of the evaluator. As a result, there are as many types of evaluation as there are evaluators. Weckwerth (1970) asks a crucial question: "Who has the right (power, influence, or authority) to decide?" He points out that "the one with the right to decide can, by specifying the what and how of evaluation, predetermine the outcome in terms of success or failure of the program" (p. 15). The singular importance of how the decision maker values the program is emphasized by several others. Ferman (1969) notes that expectations for evaluation generally vary with a person's position in the system, and Weiss (1972), following up Ferman's comment, identifies a list of persons interested in evaluation, including policymakers, program directors, practitioners, contributors, taxpayers, parents, and consumers. As she points out, evaluative questions derived from such groups will differ radically in perspective.

Another major consideration in the appraisal process is determining the purpose of an evaluation. Although authors MacMahon *et al.* (1961) and Hutchinson (1960) use different terms, they agree that evaluations can be divided into two major categories according to their underlying purposes. MacMahon *et al.* most clearly distinguish these two purposes, the first of which is to test the hypothesis that a certain practice, if successfully carried out within specified limits, has a measurable beneficial outcome in the group on whom it is practiced. This type is an "evaluation of accomplishment." The second category, "evaluations of technique," comprises studies designed to find out whether a supposedly therapeutic or preventive practice is, in fact, being carried out within specified limits. Health educators may use either or both of these to evaluate a program.

Scriven (1970) introduces the concepts of formative and summative evaluation into the discussion of purpose. In discussing the evaluation of educational curriculums, he also distinguishes between two types: formative evaluation, which produces specific information that is fed back during the development of curriculum to help improve it, thereby serving the needs of developers, and summative evaluation, which is done after the curriculum is finished in order to provide information about effectiveness to school decision makers who are considering adopting the curriculum.

Goals of Health Programs

Researchers unanimously agree that one of the most difficult and critical steps in the evaluation process is determining program goals or outcomes. Weckworth's simple operational definition of evaluation is, "Compare accomplishment with stated objectives." Difficulty arises, however, when goals are not stated or set forth in understandable terms. Indeed, evaluators may find considerable disagreement among participants where goals are concerned, as both Thorner (1972) and Elinson and Hear (1970) have convincingly shown. The major problem of abstracting goals in order to evaluate them has led to the development of two basically different approaches to evaluation: the goal-attainment model and the systems model.

The goal-attainment model views evaluation as the measurement of the degree of success or failure encountered by a program in reaching predetermined objectives. Because the model uses program goals as a yardstick to measure a program's performance, it is essential that goals be clear, specific, and measurable so that they can be translated into operational terms reflecting the consequences, or outcomes, of the program. The model is considered an objective and analytical tool because it omits the value bias of the evaluator by applying the goals of the program under study as the criteria of success. A basic assumption of this type of evaluation is that there is a relationship between a given health service and an ultimate health outcome. For example, fluoride placed in the water of a public water plant is assumed to eventually result in the reduction of tooth decay in children who drink the water. The goal-attainment model would distinguish between initial (training of personnel), intermediate (fluoride level of water), and ultimate goals (reduction in tooth decay).

A major limitation of the goal-attainment model, noted by Etzioni (1960), is that it focuses exclusively on the predetermined goals of a program. Because this limited focus does not recognize or measure other possible goals, such a model cannot explain why a program makes adaptations to its environment in order to survive. The model requires a relatively constant environment, avoids the questions of adaptation to change, and ignores the problem of perpetuation of the program itself. For example, the ultimate goal of the fluoridation program would be to reduce the rate of tooth decay in children by adding fluoride to public water systems. A major criterion used to measure the goal might be the level of fluoride in the water. If the level of fluoride were maintained at, say, .8 parts per million over a period of time, then the program would be judged successful. If not maintained, the program would be a failure. The problem is that this single criterion neither measures nor explains the variables that operate in a dynamic environment to reduce the level of fluoride in the water over a given time period. City officials might encounter public opposition to the installation of equipment, or trained operators might not be available during the first six months of the time period. If a fluoride level of .5 ppm existed initially because of such factors, such a project might be judged unsuccessful because the level of fluoride was not maintained over the fixed time period, despite the fact that the program might currently be operating successfully.

Etzioni observes that programs evaluated by the goal-attainment model invariably result in a low rating of effective performance. Because, he believes, such evaluations are artificial and frequently produce misleading conclusions, a methodological error is committed when using this model because cultural systems (i.e., goals or ideals) cannot be compared with social systems (i.e., operations or realities). Objectives that are not on the same level of analysis, he reasons, cannot be compared. Consequently, Etzioni rejects a comparison between a present state of a program (a real state) with that of a goal (an ideal state), as if the goal were also a real state. A fluoridation program that was judged unsuccessful by the goal-attainment model would probably be ruled successful by Etzioni, because he would reject a comparison of the actual level (.5 ppm) of fluoride in the water over a given time (a real state) with the goal of .8 ppm (an ideal state). Instead, he might choose goals such as the installation of equipment, training courses for operators, or, simply, the survival of the program for one year in the face of public reaction.

As an alternative to the goal-attainment model, Etzioni, Schulberg, and Baker (1968) suggest a systems model, which recognizes that organizations pursue other functions besides the achievement of predetermined (ideal state) goals. These other functions include the acquisition of resources, the coordination of subunits, and the adaptation of the organization to its environment. Returning to our example of a fluoridation program, we could identify the hiring of personnel, the training of plant operators, and the installation of equipment as functions that, according to the systems model, should be treated as part of an evaluation.

The systems model of evaluation is concerned, not simply with the achievement of goals themselves, but with the ability of an organization to establish itself as a social unit that is capable of achieving a goal. According to this model, the fluoridation project would be judged successful, because it currently has the capability of reaching the .8 ppm level of fluoride with trained plant operators and adequate equipment. According to Etzioni, "The central question in the study of effectiveness is not 'How devoted is the organization to its goal?' but rather, 'Under the given conditions, how close does the organizational allocation of resources approach an optimum distribution' " (1960, p. 258). The term *optimum* is defined as a balanced distribution of resources among the functions of organizational maintenance and goal achievement.

As we have seen, the essential difference between the goal-attainment model and the systems model is that of perspective. The goal-attainment model has a narrow perspective, focusing solely on the specific achievement of a stated goal, product, or outcome. The systems model has a much broader view, examining how a program functions at a variety of levels. It assumes that a program cannot be evaluated by a single goal or outcome. Neither can an outcome be evaluated as an entity unto itself, separate from the program that is creating it. To focus solely on such a single outcome would be unproductive and misleading. Rather, a broader perspective will reveal how a program is able to produce the outcome, survive, and improve its performance in the process.

Although we prefer the systems model, we offer a caveat: the use of this model requires more effort and expense in tracking down the specific adaptive efforts of the program to external forces that must be identified and assessed. The systems model also requires a good deal of experience to interpret findings. Finally, the suggestion that it is the best approach must be tempered by the fact that most health education programs still evaluate by the goal-attainment method.

After the goals and outcomes for a program have been determined, the next step in evaluation is to develop specific indicators or criteria to measure the extent to which the stated outcomes are achieved. The development of measures, sometimes referred to as *instrumentation,* is a demanding step.

The Development of Measurement Criteria

For health programs, this step is particularly complex because there are not adequate techniques to measure health status. To overcome this problem, three alternative approaches have been developed to measure the goals and outcomes of a program: (1) measuring whether the program has provided the intended health services, (2) measuring the objectives the health program was designed to achieve, and (3) measuring how the health program has affected the health status of the target population. The criteria for measurement differ with each approach. For example, the criteria for measuring whether health services have been provided concern the kind of structure developed to provide those services and the process by which the services were delivered. Thus, if we were to evaluate the health care services for the elderly living in a community, it would be important to determine what kind of clinics had been developed for this purpose, how accessible they were to the elderly clients, and how they were staffed. We would also want to look at the process of delivery of services: how, by whom, and when were the health services delivered to this group of people?

In the second approach, to determine whether the objectives of a program have been reached, the criteria are the impact of the program on the target population, the processes by which the objectives were achieved, and the viability of the program. (*Viability* refers to the continuing effective operation of the program.) The third approach, the assessment of how a program affects the health of the participants, relies on health status criteria: morbidity, mortality, disability, physical functioning, and social functioning. The evaluator assesses the effect of a program in terms of these measures.

Each of these approaches raises significant methodological problems regarding the appropriateness of the criteria and their validity as measures of health status. Each researcher must argue the validity of the hypothesized link between the criteria selected and health status. As a result, almost any evaluation is open to question because of the particular criteria and designs used. Further, these methodological problems, with their individual solutions, make it difficult to compare the effects of similar programs. Consequently, the development of health and social theory based on good research is hindered. Of the three approaches to the problem of measuring health in evaluation studies, the substitution of specific measures for health is probably the best accepted and most widely used. Less acceptable, but often used, are intermediate objectives, such as changes in beliefs, attitudes, or behaviors. As an approach, the least acceptable measure is that services have been provided, even though it is the most widely available single criteria.

Currently, the criteria most commonly used to measure health programs are James's (1962) set of four criteria (effort, performance, adequacy of performance, and efficiency), Hilleboe's (1968) three foci for evaluation (performance of activities, results of programs, and benefits to the community), and Roemer's (1971) adaptation of a model advanced by Donabedian (1966), which posits six criteria (costs, resources, attitudes, quantity of services, quality of services, and health status outcomes). A feature common to all these criteria is a scale, or hierarchy, ranging from low to high, with implied differences in importance. Therefore, each criterion—for example, effort—could be rated somewhere on the scale.

The Research Design

The last step in the evaluation process involves the selection of the appropriate research design and methodology needed to conduct the evaluation. This selection is crucial to the total evaluation because the research design determines the ultimate validity of the observations made about the success or failure of the program. Many evaluations have failed on methodological grounds principally because the evaluation could not separate the causal effects of program treatments from other noncausal variables.

The preferred research design is the classic experimental model. As Greenberg (1970) describes it,

> The basic design stipulates that one portion of the sampled population be allocated to the experimental treatment (i.e., the social program) and the remainder assigned to a comparison or control treatment, or placebo, and that this allocation should be done at random. After the passage of adequate time for the criterion event to develop, measurements are taken to ascertain changes in the response variables. Differences in response between the two groups are tested to determine their statistical significance before generalizing the observations for the larger population or universe (p. 165).

However, when such a design is used in an action setting involving the actual delivery of health services, a number of problems arise. The first problem concerns the allocation of different treatments to the two experimental units. As Suchman (1967) has pointed out, administrators and practitioners are understandably reluctant to withhold services from those who might benefit from them; further, it is difficult both to refuse services to those who seek them and to provide services to those who resist them. It may also be considered morally unacceptable to withhold beneficial treatment from control groups.

A second problem is that it is frequently impossible to separate the effects of program content from the characteristics of the practitioners. Staff enthusiasm and confidence can be critical variables in the success of innovative programs. When the staff is small, adjustments in design are especially difficult.

A third problem involves the reactions of program recipients. It is possible, for example, that recipients of services may contribute to the effect of an intervention through feelings of self-importance as persons selected for special attention (i.e., the Hawthorne effect) or through their faith in the program (i.e., the placebo effect).

In addition to these problems, new programs pose a special set of problems themselves. For instance, in implementing a new program, administrators frequently modify their procedures on the basis of their experiences. Such changes pose large problems if research designs call for lengthy commitment to a highly specific set of procedures. Last, some programs are diffuse and unstable. When programs involve autonomous organizations, are conducted by practitioners with professional autonomy, or are directed to uncooperative client populations, it is often necessary for evaluators to modify their designs.

As an alternative to the classic experimental design, in which participants are randomly assigned to both experimental and control groups, several authors have suggested a quasi-experimental design. The stipulation of the random assignment of participants is not possible for health educators who wish to evaluate a program that is planned to be implemented in the field. In these programs they must evaluate people who either have been selected by other criteria or have volunteered to participate. Thus, the quasi-experimental design has been developed to meet this problem and has been given some legitimacy by the work of Campbell and Stanley (1973).

All of the alternatives to the classic design involve the use of quantifiable data. As we remarked earlier, data on change are usually data reflecting change in the behavior of individuals or groups (or both). Quantitative data are usually obtained from standardized tests, questionnaire results, and cost-benefit and cost-effectiveness analyses. Because both experimental and quasi-experimental designs use data that can be measured by these instruments, these two types of designs dictate the kinds of measuring instruments that can be used and, therefore, the kind of data that can be obtained. Data on beliefs, attitudes, and values are particularly difficult to obtain by standardized measurement instruments.

What is needed is a design that will provide qualitative data. How do evaluators provide a design to obtain this kind of data? Patton (1978), exploring this problem, suggests the use of an evaluation design based on the tradition of anthropological field studies. This design aims at obtaining a detailed description of social interaction. Qualitative data consist of detailed descriptions of situations, events, people, interactions, and observed behaviors, direct quotations from people about their attitudes, beliefs, and thoughts; and excerpts from correspondence, records, and case histories.

As Patton (1980) explains this pure qualitative design, "Procedures for recruiting and selecting participants for the program are determined entirely by the staff."

The evaluator finds a convenient time to conduct an in-depth interview with participants as soon as they are admitted into the program. These in-depth interviews ask students to describe what school is like for them, what they do in school, how they typically spend their time, what their family life is like, how they approach academic tasks, their views about health, and their behaviors/attitudes with regard to delinquent and criminal activity. In brief, participants are asked to describe themselves and their social world. The evaluator finds out from program staff when the program activities will be taking place and observes those activities, collecting detailed data about what happens during those activities: participant behaviors, participant conversations, staff behaviors, staff-participant interactions, and related phenomena. During the course of the program the evaluator finds convenient opportunities for conducting additional in-depth interviews with participants to find out how they view the program, what kind of experience they are having, and what they are doing. Near the end of the program, in-depth interviews are conducted with the participants to find out what behaviors they have changed, how they view the world at this point in time, and what their expectations are for the future. In-depth interviews are also conducted with program staff. These data are content-analyzed to find out what patterns of experience participants bring to the program, what patterns characterize their participation in the program, and what patterns of change are reported by and observed in the participants (p. 112).

Quantitative and qualitative designs may be mixed. For example, an evaluator might combine qualitative measurement and content analysis or qualitative measurement and statistical analysis, or might design a naturalistic inquiry mixing qualitative measurement and statistical analysis. We believe that these mixed designs, when appropriately applied to the health education program under consideration, may provide the most effective evaluation strategy for health educators in the field of practice.

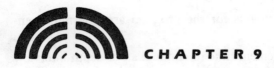

CHAPTER 9

An Analysis of Three Case Studies in Health Education

We can now examine in detail the actual practice of health education. We have selected three case studies from the recent literature, each of which deals with the theme of accident prevention among children. The first case study, "Children Can't Fly: A Program to Prevent Childhood Morbidity and Mortality from Window Falls," approaches the problem of accident prevention from a community health agency setting; the second, "Assessment of a Pilot Child Playground Injury Prevention Project in New York State," primarily uses a school setting; and the third, "Prevention of Childhood Household Injuries: A Controlled Clinical Trial," emphasizes the problem from a clinical setting.

In examining each of these three cases, we will look at five fundamental issues: (1) the relationship between setting and outcomes, and the issues of (2) planning and development, (3) organization and conduct of the program, (4) evaluation, and (5) participation. More specifically, in studying the first issue, we will be looking at the effect of an agency setting on defining problems, specifying targets for and levels of change, and determining the role of health educators. Concerning the second issue, planning and development, we will investigate how and to what extent the potential for learning opportunities within the setting was assessed, as well as the nature of the proposed educational intervention. Concerning organization and implementation, we'll want to know where the program was conducted, what personnel were involved, how it was financed, and to whom it was accountable. Pursuing our fourth issue, evaluation, we will be interested in learning the purpose of the evaluation of each program, the goals of the program, the criteria used for measuring goals, and the design of the evaluation. And, finally, we'll want to know who was involved in each aspect of the program and to what extent. We will examine the roles played by consumers, direct providers of health education, community members, decision makers, and other participants in the three programs outlined in our case studies.

C A S E   1   **Children Can't Fly: A Program to**
                          Prevent Childhood Morbidity and
                          Mortality from Window Falls

Charlotte N. Spiegel
and
Francis C. Lindaman

In a unanimous landmark decision, the New York City Board of Health on April 12, 1976, passed the first child accident prevention law of its kind in the nation. The law, an Amendment to the New York City Health Code, requires owners of multiple dwellings to provide window guards in apartments where children 10 years old and younger reside.

Enactment of the legislation ran afoul of bureaucratic and property owner resistance even though the need for this preventive legislation was documented and the deterrent prescribed. One property owner brought a proceeding in the New York State Supreme Court attacking the constitutionality of the mandate and charging *inter alia* that the Board's action shifts obligation for the care and protection of children from parents and places it on the real estate industry. However, the new regulation was upheld by the New York Supreme Court in a decision rendered by Justice Margaret J. Mangan on October 20, 1976. The court found that the Board of Health was acting within its jurisdiction granted by the New York City Charter to regulate all matters affecting health and preservation of life in New York City. The court presumed the regulation constitutional and found the action of the Board of Health "not arbitrary, capricious or unreasonable."

The genesis of this law may be traced back to a 1969 study of child mortality due to falls from heights undertaken by the New York City Department of Health for the period January 1965–September 1969. The study found that falls from heights represented 12 percent of all accidental deaths among children under 15 years of age, with window falls responsible for 123 deaths. It was recognized that mortality was only a partial perception of the problem.

Noting that 23 fall-related fatalities occurred in the South Bronx during 1971 among children 15 years or younger, the New York City Health Department initiated an education and prevention program called "Children Can't Fly" in the Tremont

Health District of the Bronx. Staff at Jacobi Hospital which served this district had recalled dozens of window falls during the previous summer, and a precinct patrolman stated that he had himself picked up nine dead children. He estimated that there were over a dozen infant deaths resulting from falls in his precinct alone every summer. Recidivism—multiple window falls in the same household—was also observed.

In the late spring of 1972 a two-year pilot program was developed combining service with research. A voluntary reporting system was initiated, and the problem of window falls was attacked through educational modalities, outreach services and the provisions of free window guards.

THE PILOT PROGRAM

The "Children Can't Fly" Program consisted of the following components:

Data Gathering

• **A Voluntary Reporting System:** Reporting of window falls of children under age 15 by police precincts and hospital emergency rooms on postal card forms supplied by the program.

• **Follow-up:** Home visits made to victim's household by public health nurses.

Education

• **One-to-One:** Outreach workers going door-to-door identifying the hazards, counseling parents on prevention, providing applications for free window guards where indicated.

• **Community Education:** Involvement of public and private agencies and community-based groups in the dissemination of prevention literature and instruction.

• **Media Campaign:** Awareness elevation and prevention education thru radio, TV, public service spot announcements, news stories, editorials, special news coverage, etc.

Prevention Service

• **Distribution of easy-to-install free window guards** to families with pre-school age children, living in tenements in high-risk areas.

This approach appeared to be effective: a downward trend in reported falls was observed by the second summer. Reported deaths from other areas indicated that the summertime epidemic of children dropping from unguarded windows continued to be one of the city's most serious accident hazards.

EXPANSION PROGRAM

In 1974 and 1975, the program was expanded to include all five boroughs. The voluntary reporting system involved contacting 63 hospital emergency rooms and 73

Table 1 / Number and Percent of Hospital Emergency Rooms and Police Precincts Participating and Reporting in Window Fall Reporting System, New York City, 1973 – 1975

	Hospitals			Precincts		
		Reporting Falls†			Reporting Falls†	
	Number Participating	No.	%	Number Participating	No.	%
1973	25	20	80	73**	15	20
1974*	45	24	53	73**	22	30
1975	63**	38	60	73**	26	36

† In children 15 years of age or younger.
* Year-round reporting initiated.
** Maximum number of hospitals with emergency room facilities.

police precincts, and periodically monitoring them on a year-round basis. It was found that if a precinct or hospital emergency room failed to report falls it usually meant that falls had not occurred within that catchment area. Personnel turnover, failure to transmit procedures from one staff person to another, and/or individual disinterest undoubtedly accounted for occasional lapses in reporting. It was useful to have both sources involved in the reporting system. Table 1 displays the growth of the program.

PUBLIC HEALTH NURSING SERVICES

The follow-up home visits made to the households of window fall victims by public health nurses were enlarged to provide supportive counseling and referral services to the victim and family. When more than this initial visit seemed indicated by conditions in the home, repeated home visits were made and appointments for clinic visits and referrals to social service agencies were arranged.

A concomitant feature of the home visit was the compilation of a report providing a family profile and demographic and sociological information. Detection and identification of other potentially dangerous environmental hazards (lead, exposed wiring, etc.) and supervisory or physical hazards (hyperactivity, mental or physical retardation, parental inability to cope) and corrective counseling were by-products of the home visit. Counseling was done on accident prevention; the family was registered for window guards and alerted to possible latent symptoms related to the accident and to the importance of clinical follow-up.

EDUCATION

The media campaign was targeted toward elevating the awareness of the public in general, and of parents in particular, to the hazard of open unguarded windows and to recommending measures for prevention of accidents. By utilizing public service time slots, special news programming, children's TV programs such as Romper Room, and capitalizing on every opportunity to issue press releases and news stories to the Spanish and English media, various agency house organs, and community papers, efforts were made to sustain the issue and the problem in the forefront of the public consciousness. Media coverage supplied the "alerting function" and presented, wherever possible, a viable solution.

Outreach workers, going door-to-door counseled on prevention; counseling was also provided in child health stations and pediatric treatment clinics. Special student trainee programs in hospital clinic waiting rooms provided another form of educational outreach.

Workshops were conducted with parents in Headstart programs and PTA groups; street programs and demonstrations were used to bring the message to a broad spectrum of the target population. There was widespread distribution of bilingual posters and multilingual flyers (English, Spanish, Chinese and Haitian) through a network of health centers, hospitals, pediatric clinics, police precincts, community councils, child health stations, family health care centers, day care centers, Headstart programs, community school boards, PTA's, child welfare agencies, offices of neighborhood services, community corporations, supermarket chains, church pastors, and a long list of community based organizations, including block associations, tenant groups, offices of community services, housing rehabilitation groups, etc.

WINDOW GUARD DISTRIBUTION

More than 16,000 free window guards were provided to approximately 4,200 families each year with particular emphasis on the high-risk areas as determined by the incidence of reported falls of the previous year, and modified by a weekly reassessment based on the most current evidence of falls in health district areas. The window guards were purchased by the New York City Health Department in open competitive bid, generally for less than $3 per guard. Environmental health personnel provided manpower for the installation of approximately 25 percent of the available guards and the remainder were distributed for self-installation. Surveys of self-installed guards were made by outreach staff to determine if guards were properly installed in appropriate windows. *There were no falls reported from windows where guards had been installed.*

PROGRAM RESULTS

The Bronx, formerly the area of highest risk, and the borough in which the "Children Can't Fly" campaign with all its components had been most intensively concen-

Table 2 / Window Fall Fatalities in Children 15 Years of Age and Under, New York City, 1973 – 1975

	Fatalities Reported by Police Precincts and Emergency Rooms	Fatalities Reported by Death Certificates			
		Total*	(a)	(b)	(c)
1973	32	57	19	2	36
1974	25	45	14	2	29
1975	19	37	10	1	26

*Includes all fatalities in children 15 years of age and younger from window falls as classified by Medical Examiner.
(a) Accidental deaths.
(b) Death where injury was purposely inflicted.
(c) Deaths where it is undetermined if injury was purposely inflicted.

trated, has remained relatively constant in the number of reporting agencies participating since the inception of the program. In the Bronx 108 falls were reported in 1973, declined to 64 in 1974, and to 54 in 1975, a 50 percent decline in two years. During the critical summer months of June-September 1973–1975, a highly significant decline in reported falls was recorded: the percentage decline was 50 percent in September 1975 as compared with the same months in 1973, 68 percent in June, 72.8 percent in July, and 81.5 percent in August.

City-wide, in 1973, there were 192 falls reported. In 1974, the number reported was 132, a decrease of 31 percent. In 1975, 159 falls were reported, a 20 percent increase over 1974. However, between 1974 and 1975 the number of reporting emergency rooms increased from 24 to 38.

Given the potential for errors of omission and commission possible in a voluntary reporting system in the reporting of falls, deaths may be a better barometer. The number of deaths of children due to falls from heights in the city as determined from death certificates declines from 57 in 1973 to 45 in 1974 and to 37 in 1975, a decrease of 35 percent since 1973. These data are displayed in Table 2.

Selected data taken from the reports of falls are tabulated in Table 3. Male victims exceed females in a 2.1 ratio; children fell from bedroom windows with greater frequency than from other rooms; and more falls occurred during the afternoon hours than at any other time of the day.

It is difficult to assign a primary cause to most accidents since many factors contribute to the occurrence. For example, a child left alone in a room may also have climbed on furniture to reach a window, and may have opened a window that had been closed. The same child may or may not have been the victim of neglect, or the parent may have assumed that the child was asleep and in no danger. Cultural or environmental factors such as the use of fire escapes as sitting or play areas play their

Table 3 / Selected Characteristics of Victims of Window Falls Reported* February-October, 1973 – 1975, New York City

Characteristics	No.	%
Total reported falls	483	100.0
Sex		
Male	322	67
Female	161	33
Age		
0 – 2 yrs.	160	33.3
3 – 5 yrs.	186	38.5
6 – 15 yrs.	137	28.2
Ethnicity		
Black	194	40.1
Hispanic	247	51.1
Other	42	8.8
Economic support		
Welfare	244	50.5
Parent employed	178	36.9
Unknown	61	12.6
Month of occurrence		
February	4	0.8
March	9	1.9
April	17	3.5
May	40	8.3
June	94	19.5
July	150	31.1
August	93	19.2
September	52	10.7
October	24	4.9
Time of day		
Morning	93	19.2
Afternoon	219	45.4
Evening	156	32.3
Unknown	15	3.1
Location of occurrence		
Bedroom	119	25
Living room	123	25.3
Kitchen	69	14.2
Other (fire escapes, etc.)	77	15.6
Unknown	77	15.6
Roof	21	4.3
Circumstances surrounding fall		
Alone in room	224	46.4
Horseplay	138	28.6
Faulty screens	67	13.8
Foul play (suicide, homicide, neglect, abuse)	25	5.2
Unknown	29	6.0

*As reported by police precincts and hospital emergency rooms.

parts, since children may climb out of windows in order to sit or play in these areas and then fall.

A majority of falls occurred in single parent households and approximately 60 percent of the families were supported by social services in 1975 as compared with 37 percent in 1973. This latter increase may be a reflection of the worsening economic conditions.

Since approximately 90 percent of falls occur from tenement type buildings, which do not make up 90 percent of the city's housing stock, an association exists between the incidence of falls and environmental factors such as aging or deteriorating housing. The hazard of falls from buildings in the same age category is not diminished where construction is no higher than three stories, although fatalities are fewer. There is an association between incidence of falls and the economically disadvantaged since it is this group that resides in substandard housing under circumstances of overcrowding, family instability, tensions, and pressures.

DISCUSSION

Medicaid payment for inpatient care in New York City is currently over $200 per diem. For the two-year period 1974–1975, the cost of inpatient treatment for victims of window falls—excluding emergency room diagnoses and treatment, after-care, rehabilitation and maintenance—was calculated at $544,904 for 170 known cases admitted to hospitals.

The 1975 list of casualties, aside from fatalities, includes cases of children who sustained brain damage, paralysis, loss of kidneys, ruptured spleens and bladders, loss of eyesight, and similar incapacitating injuries which portend extended if not permanent after-care and maintenance, the dollar cost of which has not been included or projected as a cost factor in the above estimate.

These reasons, together with the evidence provided by the voluntary program described above led to the amendment of the Health Code of the City of New York in April, 1976. This mandate will be incrementally implemented according to a three-year phase-in plan in which the high-risk areas are required to comply in the first year, the moderate risk areas in the second year, and the remainder of the city by March 31, 1979.

The office of Professional and Public Health Education of the Health Department will continue its educational efforts and inform property owners of their obligations under the Health Code regulation. It will educate the public, particularly parents, about their entitlements under the mandated timetable, and will instruct and assist tenants in notifying property owners of their family composition relative to children in the affected age category, to establish their eligibility for receiving the window guards, and to expedite compliance with the regulation.

The incidence of fatalities from window falls among children in New York City alone approximates the nationwide data for aspirin poisoning fatalities which precipitated the passage of federal accident prevention legislation. Whereas no data are currently available relevant solely to the incidence of window falls and fatalities nationally, it may be assumed that falls occur and fatalities result in large urban areas wherever there are conditions of low socioeconomic population, deteriorating housing, overcrowding, family instability, etc. Therefore, one preventive health education module and service program based on this type of campaign and the legislation that evolved therefrom might serve as a useful prototype.

CASE 2   **Assessment of a Pilot Child Playground Injury Prevention Project in New York State**

Leslie Fisher, Virginia Goddard Harris, John VanBuren, John Quinn, and Alison DeMaio

During 1978 data from the National Electronic Injury Surveillance System (NEISS), a statistically representative sampling of hospitals with emergency departments, projected that about 155,500 playground-related injuries—almost equally divided between home and public playgrounds—were treated in emergency departments nationwide. There had been 118,000 such injuries in 1974.

The predominant playground accident was falls; major injuries included strangulations, concussions, amputations, fractures, contusions, dislocations, sprains, and lacerations. Ninety-three percent of playground injuries were incurred by children under 15 years of age.

Because of the variety of playground users and equipment, the diverse way the equipment may be used, and the many nonequipment factors involved in overall playground safety, mandatory equipment specifications by themselves cannot adequately address the problem.

We organized and executed a pilot playground accident prevention program in 1977–78. The program and efforts to measure its impact are described.

MATERIALS AND METHODS

During the fall of both 1977 and 1978 we conducted a total of 30 standardized, 40-minute workshops for 1,500 professional leaders involved in the purchase, installation, maintenance, and supervision of public playgrounds. Recreational leaders, day care centers and elementary school teachers, nurses, and parent/teacher representatives participated. These workshops offered new knowledge for motivating voluntary correction at minimal cost of obvious equipment hazards. Factual materials were distributed, and the CPSC film, "Swing That Swing Back," was shown and discussed. Pre- and post-tests measured changes in participant's knowledge.

In addition, more than 60 Consumer Deputies* (unpaid volunteers from among local parent-teacher associations, consumer groups, women's groups and school teachers) attended our half-day orientation-training seminars on the purpose of the project, and the nature and extent of playground-equipment injuries. We also conducted, for the deputies, role-playing exercises to identify and offer suggestions for voluntary correction following playground surveys, using a CPSC survey-checklist of 12 observable, easily correctable hazards.**

A public informational phase was conducted, using radio public service announcements and newspaper articles, to convey messages to parents with backyard playground equipment. Public exhibits about playground safety, staged in shopping centers and at fairs, featured quiz boards, puppet shows, and "talking" unsafe playground equipment. We also distributed approximately 50,000 playground safety leaflets and coloring books to the general public.

In 1977, we randomly surveyed 110 playgrounds operated by the schools, municipalities, and state and local park systems. These surveys, done by the trained consumer deputies and our site coordinators (educators or sanitarians), were repeated in 1978.

In both years we relied upon the CPSC survey-checklist of hazards. Many hazards, easily correctable by temporarily taping surfaces or tightening parts, were voluntarily corrected at minimal cost.

RESULTS

Playground personnel taking the pre- and post-tests at the first three workshops in each site in 1978 increased their correct scores by 17 percent (Table 1). At the Syracuse site, only three persons had all answers correct at pre-test, while 36 persons did at post-test.

Table 2 shows a 42 percent reduction in 1978 in observed average number of hazards per playground site compared to 1977. For example, in Monroe County in 1978 hard surfaces were observed in only nine (26 percent) of the playgrounds, compared to 24 (71 percent) in 1977; such surfaces are usually associated with the most

---

*As an unpaid volunteer, the consumer deputy, under supervision of a health professional, had no authority to order changes, but he/she did record risks and promote voluntary correction of observed possible risks in communal playground equipment. This limited the need of professional inspector staff for initial surveillance. For further information on the use of Consumer Deputies, request fact sheet #80, The Consumer Deputy Program, from CPSC, Washington, DC 20207. Deputies have been used to voluntarily survey homes, retail stores, and public places for unsafe surroundings, practices or products.

**Sharp edges; underlying hard surfaces (e.g., concrete, brick, blacktop); sharp or piercing crushing points; inadequate spacing (less than six feet away from obstructions); open hooks; loose and protruding bolts; hard, heavy seats; loose anchoring; and parts that could entrap—by equipment type (e.g., swings, slides, seesaws).

Table 1 / Pre- and Post-Test Scores of Participants in 1978 Workshops

Test Site	No. of Seminars	Estimated No. in Audience	No. of People Tested*	Overall Pre-Score	Overall Post-Score	Percent Improvement**
				%	%	%
Syracuse	6	149	69	83	96	+ 13
Rochester	3	47	31	65	90	+ 25
Totals	9	196	100	77	94	+ 17

*People tested in each site were attendees of the first three seminars. Workshops were not conducted in Suffolk nor Albany test sites in 1978.
**A difference of means test was conducted and the percent improvement was statistically significant at the $p < 0.05$ level in each instance.

Table 2 / Comparisons of Playgrounds Surveys, 1977 – 1978*

	Number Surveys Repeated in 1977 & 1978	Average No. Hazards/Playground Site**		Percent Reduction Observed in Average No. Hazards/Playground Site
		1977	1978	
				%
Albany	17	16.76	8.17	– 51
Rochester	34	8.32	5.44	– 35
Syracuse	23	3.78	2.35	– 38
Total	74	8.85	5.11	– 42

* Of the 108 playgrounds surveyed in 1977, 74 (70 percent) were resurveyed in 1978 where school officials could first be contacted.
** Only playgrounds surveyed in both 1977 and 1978 are included in average hazard/playground.

serious injuries from falls. In Onondaga County, many heavy swing seats observed in 1977 were replaced with lighter canvas.

The only available injury frequency data, derived from the NEISS system for Rochester's two largest hospitals, indicated that there were 22.4 percent fewer injuries treated or treated and admitted to those hospitals in July–December, 1977 and 1978, than in the same period of 1975 and 1976 (average of 97 vs. 125). Table 3 shows the trend through 1978. In 1979, the Consumer Product Safety Commission redesigned the NEISS system and these two hospitals were excluded.

Table 3 / Injuries Associated with Playground Equipment among
All Age Groups, Reported to NEISS System: Rochester, N.Y.,
Rochester General and Strong Memorial Hospitals (Treatment Dates
July 1 – December 31, 1975, and 1978)

Recorded Period, July 1 – Dec. 31	Injuries Reported	Percent Change from Previous Year
1975	149	—
1976	101	– 32.2
1977	73	– 27.7
1978	120	64.4

Average injuries over intervention period (1977 – 78)	97	
Percent reduction vs. base years (1975 – 76)	$\dfrac{125 - 97 \times 100}{125} = 22.4$	

Source of data National Injury Information Clearinghouse, NEISS Data Detail, CPSC,
Washington, DC.

DISCUSSION

While the results of these inexpensive efforts are encouraging, the project can only
be considered as a pilot effort. The apparent decrease in injuries treated in only two
hospitals in one project site is not sufficient proof of program effectiveness. Similarly,
our analysis of playground risks from specific playground equipment was limited by
the CPSC designed survey-checklist. The shortcomings of the survey-checklist included the inability to record actual numbers of specific types of equipment, e.g., a
playground with multi-swing sets or slides is treated the same as a playground with
only one swing set or slide. Furthermore, a swing set with multiple sharp edges was
treated the same as a swing set with only one sharp edge. Finally, the data do not
explore long-term effects of the program. Nonetheless, the collected data do give an
overall impression of various indices of improved outcomes associated with the pilot
project.

Health professionals must begin to translate data about the nature and extent of
child injuries into active empirically based preventive programs for reductions in unsafe behavior, risks, and injury, followed by program evaluation efforts. Moreover,
such preventive efforts will also help limit the need for expensive medical care programs. Many "proximate solutions" appear possible.

C A S E 3

Prevention of Childhood Household Injuries: A Controlled Clinical Trial

Robert A. Dershewitz
and
John W. Williamson

INTRODUCTION

Accidents claim more lives of children between ages one and 15 than the next six leading pediatric disorders combined. As many as one out of every three children each year will require medical attention for injuries and, among pediatric acute illnesses, accidents are second in frequency only to respiratory disease. Ninety-one percent of all injuries to children under five years of age occurred at home, and more than one-half of all fatal injuries to preschoolers occur in and around the home.

Prevention of childhood accidents is of great importance to both individuals and society but, unfortunately, has largely been either excluded from attention or treated in an inappropriate manner. Adequate countermeasures for dealing with those preventable aspects of injury control are poorly understood and much in need of study.

The purpose of this project was to develop and evaluate an effective method of reducing the risk of childhood household injuries. Educational attention to those hazards shown in the literature to be most in need of reduction was the focus of a practical model designed to deal with this problem.

METHODS

Study Design

An experimental design based on Campbell and Stanley's "post-test only" control group design was used. As applied here, this design involved participation of a consecutive group of mothers seeking care for their preschool children in a prepaid health plan clinic. These mothers were randomly allocated to an experimental and a control group. The experimental group participated in a personalized health education program to effect reduction of household hazards. One month after completion of the health education program, both experimental and control groups received an unannounced household hazard assessment and survey questionnaire by a home visitor who was unaware of whether the mother belonged to the experimental or control group. The two groups of mothers were compared with respect to their knowledge, attitudes, and behavior related to the health problem of household accidents. Using this design, significant differences could be attributed to the experimental variable, namely the educational program.

The study population were members of the prepaid Columbia Medical Plan (CMP) in the new planned city of Columbia, Maryland, located approximately mid-way between Baltimore and Washington, D.C. Data from a 1973 survey indicated that about 90 percent of the household heads attended college, 81 percent of the household heads were white, and the median household annual income was $19,000.

Currently, approximately 38 percent of the population are members of the CMP with 70 percent of the enrollees under 35 years of age and 8.6 percent under age 5. The types and frequency of injuries in this latter group were comparable to other published series from other middle class groups, even though the socioeconomic and demographic characteristics of the study group were above the national average.

After the child completed his medical visit at the CMP, consecutive eligible mothers were asked to stop by the office of the research assistant of the project before leaving the medical building. Mothers with children who were acutely ill, had chronic debilitating illnesses, behavioral disorders, or who were presented for preoperative clearance were excluded from participation in the study. This was intended to minimize the stress of the medical visit, thereby enabling the mother to be more attentive and receptive to the safety intervention. The research assistant told mothers that (1) participation was entirely voluntary; (2) an unannounced home inspection might be requested at some future time; and (3) if safety hazards were present, recommendations would be offered to correct this situation and in no way would deficiencies at home be used to the detriment of the mother.

Upon agreeing to participate in the project, the mothers were assigned to either an experimental (E) or control (C) group through the use of a table of random numbers. For those assigned to the E group, the first stage of a two-stage educational intervention was begun. This first stage lasted approximately 20 minutes and consisted of two approaches:

1. The research assistant discussed with the mothers the most significant problem areas in household safety relevant to the age of her child. Important risk factors that were most likely to result in an injury to the child as well as anticipatory counseling were covered. A didactic lecture was avoided by encouraging the mother to be as active as possible in this session by exploring such areas as past injury experience and perceived benefits and barriers to preventive action. Common misbeliefs such as "most accidents cannot be avoided" were also addressed.

2. A booklet, designed for this project, entitled "10 Ways in 10 Days for Making Your Child Safer" was given to each mother in the experimental group. This booklet was comprehensive in providing specific recommendations to the mother for eliminating a broad range of common household child health hazards, and encouraged the mother to take active responsibility in utilizing this resource. She was instructed to work through one page of the ten-page booklet each day. Each page concentrated on one type of home injury, e.g., burns, falls, etc. The overall format was a brief

exposition of the daily theme in concrete terms, followed by a check-off list with specific, practical recommendations for the mother to follow to prevent future burns, falls, etc.

Before leaving the clinic, each mother was given, free of charge, a packet of eight electric outlet covers and three kindergards, which are easily installed plastic locking devices intended to prevent children from getting into cabinets.

The second and final stage of the educational intervention, presented to the experimental group about four weeks after the initial encounter by the same research assistant, consisted of a telephone call in which the mothers were questioned as to their involvement in the project and difficulties they incurred while trying to follow the recommendations regarding household hazard reduction. If the mother stated she had not complied with the recommendations in the booklet, the research assistant reviewed the initial discussion with emphasis on importance and motivation, to ascertain any difficulties in completing any of the tasks. If the mother had successfully completed the programmed assignment, positive reinforcement was given, and the mother was told that her child would be sent a coloring book which stressed household safety.

Approximately four weeks after the completion of the second stage, an unannounced home visit was randomly made to a sample of approximately 100 from each of the E and C groups. The home visitor had not previously participated in the project, and was not told which family belonged to which group. Thus, the home evaluation was performed in as blind a manner as possible.

At the same time, a questionnaire designed to ascertain the mother's knowledge, beliefs, and behavior regarding home injury control was administered to both the E and C groups. Every item of the questionnaire was specifically covered at least once during the safety education. Although this instrument was compiled for this study, it was based on existing behavior prevention questionnaires which had undergone previous validity and reliability testing.

The Household Hazard Scale

The instrument used for obtaining the dependent variable (i.e., hazards) was based on two factors: (1) degree of exposure as determined by the home inspector; and (2) degree of potential injury severity, a numerical value derived from the National Electronic Injury Surveillance System (NEISS) statistics for 1975. In this system, each hazard is rated by its unique "Mean Severity Score," based on the frequency a hazard is associated with a given injury weighted by the potential severity of that injury. The extent of exposure was judged on a scale of 1–3, where 1 indicated that the given hazard was not present, 2 represented one or two hazards exposed in the home, and 3 meant three or more hazards were exposed in the home.

Eleven potential hazards, each covered in the safety booklet, were arbitrarily selected for evaluation. Each of these 11 items (see Table 2, p. 179) had a final score formulated by multiplying the degree of exposure by its logarithmically transformed mean severity score (in order to normalize the means). The individual final scores were added, yielding a cumulative safety index for each home. The higher the score, the greater were the existing hazards. The scale, as applied in this study, achieved an inter-observer reliability pre-test of 83 percent.

RESULTS

Of the 330 consecutive mothers eligible to participate in the project, only 22 declined to participate, giving a consent rate of 93.3 percent. The youngest child in most (approximately 75 percent) of the participating families was under three years of age. During the project, only three (0.9 percent) dropped out, all at the time of the home visit. Initially, each group had approximately 150 members. During the four months of the data collection, several families moved and were then dropped from the study. Of those remaining eligible, 101 from the E group and 104 from the C group were arbitrarily chosen for final outcome measurements.

Table 1 shows that both groups were comparable in those sociodemographic variables thought to be most relevant. As a non-parametric analysis in Table 2 illustrates, there was a quantitatively similar hazard exposure for both groups. The fact that no differences at the $p = .05$ level were revealed permitted the data to be expressed in the manner shown in Table 3. Use of the Household Hazard Scale reveals that there is no difference in final scores, both in the number of individual hazards and in the total household safety scores for each of the 11 items mentioned in the safety booklet.

Data from the questionnaire revealed that of the 101 mothers in the E group, only four completed all the recommendations in the safety booklet, 71 completed some of the safety proofing, and 22 mothers did not use the booklet.

Table 4 addresses the issue of possible discrepancies between answers to questions which ask if the hazard is present, and its actual presence as determined by the home inspector. Since correlations were done only on those four items presented in Table 4, conclusions regarding the reliability of responses are tentative. Mothers were inaccurate in reporting the presence or absence of cleaning materials under the kitchen sink, but answers become highly correlated in response to questions related to the presence of kitchen knives, matches, lighters, and electric outlet covers.

In all instances, answers on the questionnaire revealed no difference in accident-related preventive behavior and knowledge of household accidents. Thus the interest that most mothers in the E group claimed to have had in the project did not relate to subsequent preventive behavior. The educational program also had little effect on belief, except for one item in which the experimental mothers *thought* that their homes were safer as a result of their participation in the study. Direct observation proved this to be a misperception.

DISCUSSION

Because of problems of prevalence, feasibility, and multiple variables, the presence of household hazards was used as a proxy measure of injuries. Literature review provides research support for a linkage between a reduction of hazards and a reduction of injuries. For example, it has been well demonstrated that child-resistant con-

Table 1 / Comparison of Characteristics of the Experimental and Control Groups

	Experimental	Control	Std Dev	P value using x^2	Significance
	(N = 101)	(N = 104)			
Age of mother	median = 30 yrs.	median = 30 yrs.	4.2	0.54	NS
Work status of mother	85% unemployed	76% unemployed	0.6	0.25	NS
Number of children per family	median = 2	median = 2	0.8	0.66	NS
Marital status	100% married	99% married	0.1	0.25	NS
Type of dwelling	91% lived in house or townhouse	97% lived in house or townhouse	0.6	0.11	NS
Duration of membership in the Columbia Medical Plan	median = 30 mo.	median = 34 mo.	22.97	0.31	NS

Table 2 / Number of Homes Having Specified Quantity of Observed Hazards

Type of Hazard	None*		1–2**		3 or more***	
	Experimental	Control	Experimental	Control	Experimental	Control
Cleaning agents	1	0	7	9	93	95
Prescription drugs	22	20	34	38	45	45
Waxes and polishes	51	40	44	57	5	5
Nonprescription drugs	1	3	12	16	88	85
Coins	30	47	27	18	44	37
Jewelry, watches, keys	13	14	41	45	47	45
Appliances on counter tops	2	4	76	77	23	23
Matches exposed	47	43	27	34	27	26
Pins and needles	33	31	36	33	32	38
Kitchen knives	32	38	38	34	30	30
Hazards on floor	69	72	19	16	12	13

*Hazard not present.

**1 or 2 hazards exposed in the home.

***3 or more hazards exposed in the home.

Note: Wilcoxin Rank Sum Test comparing experimental and control groups revealed no statistically significant differences at the $p = .05$ level.

Table 3 / Item Analysis of Presence of Hazard Determined on Home Visit.*

	Experimental (Mean) N = 101	Control (Mean) N = 104
Cleaning agents	8.73	8.74
Prescription drugs	6.68	6.73
Waxes and polishes	4.64	5.01
Nonprescription drugs	8.55	8.37
Coins	6.38	5.73
Jewelry, watches, keys	4.67	4.60
Appliances on counter tops	4.42	4.35
Matches exposed	3.60	3.70
Pins and needles	2.00	2.15
Kitchen knives	2.03	2.02
Hazards on floor	1.50	1.59
Total household hazard scores	53.20	52.99

*Refer to text for explanation of scale.
Note: Use of student's t = test revealed nonsignificant differences at the p = .05 level.

---

tainers can prevent poisoning; placing slats closer together on cribs can prevent strangulation; banning dangerous toys can reduce the incidence of toy-induced injuries; and protecting children from space heaters and open fireplaces can reduce accidental burns. Indeed, a near consensus of expert opinion is reflected in the final report of the National Commission on Product Safety: "A significant number of accidents could have been spared if more attention had been paid to hazard reduction."

There are divergent theories of the best approach to injury control, but most strategies incorporate, to varying degrees, the need for modification of human behavior through health education. Difficulties at arriving at a unified approach include the multiplicity of dynamic variables involved as well as the confounding observation that what works for some patients and problems does not work for all.

Some investigators stress the importance of more intensive and comprehensive management of the "accident repeater." Although this strategy may be appropriate in certain individual situations, it would not seem to be cost-effective as a leading countermeasure in injury control since repeaters and accident prone children represent only a small minority of at-risk children. From April 1975 to March 1976, less than 2 percent of the children enrolled in the CMP had more than two reported injuries of any type.

Other investigators advocate passive measures as the best approach and recommend legislation for mandatory safety standards. The two most cogent arguments for this approach are: (1) the manifest effectiveness (e.g., safety caps on medicine bottles prevent many ingestions); and (2) a lesser need for individual action and responsibility, both of which are very difficult to motivate.

Table 4 / Mothers' Responses on the Questionnaire Correlated with the Actual Presence of the Hazard as Determined by the Home Inspector

		Hazard Observed by Inspector							
		Cleaning Agents Under Sink		Kitchen Knives on Kitchen Counter		Matches/Lighters Lying Around House		Usage of Electric Outlet Covers	
		Present*	Absent	Present	Absent	Present	Absent	Present	Absent
Hazard Perceived by Mother									
Experimental	Yes	53	1	20	3	37	7	38	1
	No	47	0	47	29	19	40	41	11
	Level of significance**	$P = .31$		$p = .05$		$p < .001$		$p < .01$	
Control	Yes	61	0	11	7	37	11	48	5
	No	40	0	51	30	21	32	38	15
	Level of significance**	$P = 1.0$		$p < .001$		$p < .001$		$p < .05$	

* Since the purpose of the table is to show discrepancies, the presence of any number of hazards is recorded as being present.

** The Kappa Statistic, although not widely used, is the most appropriate test to use when correlations are examined (29).

Still other investigators stress innovative health education approaches as an effective means of improving patient behavior. However, too often in practice, "education" has been operationalized as mass dissemination of information and platitudes by such means as pamphlets, films, and displays.

Why did the educational intervention used in this study fail so completely? Since Columbia, Maryland, is hardly an average city, could the home safety practices there be exceptionally high? After the data were collected, this possibility was tested by having the same home visitor make an unannounced visit to ten random homes located in middle class communities in Baltimore and in a rural town in Pennsylvania. The home hazard scores of these ten homes (mean of 53.0) were comparable to that of the study sample, suggesting that the issue of generalizability was not a significant problem in this study.

In those instances in which health education has been shown to be effective, there was usually a well-defined target population and the thrust was to modify a single focused behavior. In the current study, on the other hand, many behaviors were required to be changed simultaneously. Consequently, both the impact of the message and expectancy of the action were likely diluted. Thus health education is less likely to be effective when applied to as broad a field as household injury control. Even if the study were successful in terms of a more restricted goal such as electric burn prevention by the use of electric outlet covers, it is doubtful whether all household accidents would have been reduced significantly.

Another important finding relates to the credibility and method of evaluation. Most outcome studies of this nature have used only written or verbal responses and accepted their accuracy. However, if correlation between the reporting and the actual "in vivo situation" is absent or erratic, then both the choice of evaluative methodology and the validity of the interpretation may be suspect. The fact that the E group mothers believed that their homes were safer as a result of their participation in the study was either a misperception or an attempt to respond in a way they thought was expected of them. Whatever the reason, it serves to replicate similar alterations of self-perceived actions found in other studies. This study also revealed inconsistencies in the reporting of hazards on questionnaires. The explanation of why the misperception was limited to only cleaning agents under the sink remains obscure.

Another health education strategy, or a shift of emphasis in the one employed, might have been more successful. Although unlikely to have had important bearing on the results, several other potential methodologic problems should be mentioned: (1) dissemination of the safety message from the E group to the C group; (2) extraneous intervening variables; (3) validity of the Household Hazard Scale; and (4) the "post-test only" experimental design might have masked differences in baseline measurements.

IMPLICATIONS

National and local health workers should use approaches which seem to have the greatest potential payoff. In the field of injury control, passive measures such as well-conceived construction and product safety regulations are more effective than attempts at changing human behavior. Spending hundreds of millions of dollars to broadcast ineffective health messages and platitudes, as has happened so often in the past, hardly seems worthwhile. New approaches should be evaluated on a demonstration basis prior to widescale implementation. This strategy seems self-evident, but probably most health education campaigns in the past have been carried out before their effectiveness had been established. In any event, for many injury control areas, the strategy with the greatest chance for success is one in which a modification in behavior is minimized. It is the "passive measures" approach that should receive most attention both in current emphasis and future research.

An Analysis of the Three Cases

Needs Assessment of the Setting

The first essential competency of a health educator is the ability to understand a setting in relation to its external environment. The setting defines the problem by defining targets for change and levels of change as well as specifying roles of the change agent. Table 9.1 presents an analysis of each of the three cases using these dimensions (see pp. 184–85).

The table makes it quite clear that the prepaid clinical setting in Case 3 has, by its nature, limited the scope of its needs assessment. Consequently, the targets and levels of change in Case 3 were limited to parents, in contrast to the direct providers, community agencies, and decision makers that a public health agency setting would have involved. In contrast, a needs assessment for Case 1, which took a more comprehensive approach, emphasized not only more targets but also levels of change, including second-order macro change. Clearly, a community setting can allow for a greater diversity of change options than other settings. In a similar manner, the role of the change agent was greater in Case 1 because of the extensive community orientation of its program. Change agents in Cases 2 and 3 were more limited in their narrow focus.

Plan and Program Development

The second essential competency of a health educator is the ability to design an educational intervention appropriate for a specific setting. Table 9.2 (see pp. 186–87) lists variables that are integral to plan development. It shows that the success of any planned intervention begins with an assessment of the learning opportunities that could potentially occur in a given setting; the assessment must consider not only the setting but also the timing, the educator, and the learner to be involved. The opportunities for learning in Cases 1 and 2 were greater than in Case 3 because of the greater number of settings where learning opportunities could occur. Case 3 was self-limiting, due to its single setting. Thus, we see that the success

Table 9.1 *Needs Assessment of the Settings* (Cases 1, 2, and 3)

	Case 1	Case 2	Case 3
A. Agency setting	Large urban public health departments	State public health agency (limited to school focus)	Prepaid health plan, clinical setting
B. Definition of problem	High incidence of mortality and morbidity associated with falls from windows	High incidence of morbidity and mortality linked to unsafe playground practices and equipment hazards	High incidence of injuries occurring in the home (burns, falls, etc.)
C. Targets for change	1. Parents of children under 5 years old 2. Landlords 3. Direct providers (hospitals, police) 4. Community agencies 5. Decision makers	1. Parents of children under 15 years old 2. Playground supervisors 3. Community groups (P.T.A.'s, consumer groups, school teachers) 4. Professional leaders and decision makers (involved in purchase and installation of playground equipment)	Parents of pre-school age children

D. Levels of change	1. First-order micro change (counseling parents) 2. First-order macro change installing window guards and conducting educational programs) 3. Second-order macro change (passage of law requiring window guards)	1. First-order micro change (public information programs for parents) 2. First-order macro change (correcting hazards and establishing of surveillance system)	First-order micro change (educational program for parents to correct existing hazards in homes)
E. Role of change agent	1. Coordinate community-wide program 2. Supervise outreach 3. Facilitate community groups 4. Advocate regulation	1. Coordinate community-wide program 2. Facilitate workshops	1. Educate parents 2. Supervise follow-up evaluation

Table 9.2 *Plan and Program Development* (Cases 1, 2, and 3)

	Case 1	Case 2	Case 3
A. Assessment of learning opportunities			
1. Setting	Home, hospitals, clinics, community agencies, media, legislature	Schools, playgrounds, and local communities	Clinic
2. Timing	Summer months (associated with high incidence)	Early in school year	After a regular clinic visit
3. Educator	Outreach worker, direct providers, health educators, community leaders	Health educators, "consumer deputies," public health workers, school personnel	Research assistant
4. Learner	Parents, community leaders, landlords, legislators, direct providers	Parents, professional leaders, teachers, community groups	Parents of preschool age children
B. Assessment of existing learning opportunities within setting			
1. Quantity and distribution of LO's	Not known	Not known	Not known
2. Quality of LO's	Not known	Not known	Not known
3. Continuity of LO's	Not known	Not known	Not known

4. Efficiency of LO's	Not known	Not known	Not known
5. Nature of proposed educational intervention			
a) Group in need	Specific neighborhoods inhabited by a lower economic group, mainly on welfare and including a high percentage of blacks and Hispanics. Main target: children under 5	Recreational supervisors and parents of children using public playgrounds	Mothers of preschool children (highly educated, white, high median income)
b) Objectives	Change behavior of family members and children; change behavior of household so window guards are placed; create community awareness on need for community action; influence decision makers to support safety regulation	Change knowledge and attitudes of persons attending workshops; change behavior of parents; change behavior of playground supervisors until hazards are corrected	Change behavior of mothers supervising children; change existing household hazards
c) Methods	Major elements included: reporting system, followup; one to one and community education; media campaign; installation of window guards	Workshops providing new knowledge; use of PTA volunteers called "consumer deputies"; media campaign; health-hazard reporting system	One-on-one discussion; printed material; free payment of safety services; follow-up telephone call with mailed printed material
d) Evaluation	Change in frequency of window falls and number of related fatalities	Pre- and post-test scores of participants and reduction of observed hazards	Assessment of: hazards in household; knowledge, beliefs, and behaviors (of mothers)

of a health education program is related to the number of settings where learning opportunities may occur.

Timing is a crucial factor in the determination of the learning opportunities. In Cases 1 and 2, the timing was especially appropriate because the program was linked to seasonal incidence of the problem. In contrast, the intervention in Case 3 was integrated into a regular clinic visit and therefore not related to a specific event. Educational principles suggest that learners are more receptive when what is being taught (the content) can be directly related to their own recent experience.

It is important that health educators clearly distinguish who can teach (the educator) and who, specifically, is the learner. Case 1 defined the educator in the most comprehensive fashion; a variety of people were involved in the educational role. Case 2 was more limited by focusing on school personnel, playground supervisors, and "consumer deputies." In Case 3, the educator was defined simply as the teacher, which overlooked the educational roles of doctors, nurses, and other clinic personnel. Because the program planners did not involve these other health professionals as educators, the potential number of learning opportunities that could potentially have been provided the learner was reduced. In contrast, Case 1 utilized the "teaching-learning-teaching process" that is basic to health education theory. In this instance, the theory and principles of the problem were taught to community leaders who, in turn, became the educators.

After assessing the potential for learning opportunities in a given setting, it is important to assess the existing learning opportunities in the setting, identifying their number and rating their effectiveness. In each of our three cases, this information is not available perhaps, because the authors of the case descriptions failed to mention any existing learning opportunities, or because an assessment was simply not done. In any event, such an assessment is essential in order to be able to establish baseline measurement.

The final step in the program development sequence is the design of an educational intervention which we referred to in Chapter 5 as the preparation of the plan, or the statement of needs, objectives, methods, and evaluation. First, the learners and their needs must be specifically identified. It is important to involve learners at this point in order to identify their knowledge, attitudes, and beliefs about the problem. This information is then used to write appropriate objectives, on which the intervention is based. Next, methods to implement these objectives are established. Finally, an evaluation is designed that will measure objectives and determine if the intervention was successful.

In Case 1, needs assessment began with the development of an elaborate reporting system that identified all window falls in the target area. Each accident was investigated by a public health nurse in order to determine characteristics associated with its occurrence. Program objectives were developed using a profile of the victims; these objectives emphasized behavioral change in all those families with children under five years of age (i.e., potential victims) and also dealt with organizational change of the environment (i.e., installation of window guards). A number of methods were used, including a reporting system, follow-up cases, parental counseling, community education, use of media, and free installation of window guards. An unusual part of this case was the ongoing use of evaluation to reshape the program. New information obtained from continued evaluation resulted in expansion of the program and provided the necessary groundwork for passage of a law. Case 1 is thus an excellent example of how evaluation can form a feedback loop to improve the program design.

In contrast to the first case, needs assessment in Case 2 stressed a different aspect of the problem. Instead of emphasizing playground injuries and exploring their occurrence within a target population, the planners in Case 2 chose to survey all playgrounds to determine possible hazards. By focusing on equipment rather than children, they arrived at objectives that would reduce the number of hazards. Linking these objectives to methods, they then developed workshops for playground directors, supervisors, and teachers. In this instance the behavioral change was directed toward decision makers (those who had the power to alter the playground environment), rather than potential victims. "Consumer deputies" were also organized to survey playgrounds within the target area, and knowledge tests were used to measure behavioral change among program participants. At the conclusion of the program the playground hazards survey was repeated.

The Case 3 planners did not begin their program with a needs assessment. Rather, they based their needs on assumptions derived from national data on household injuries to children. Little or no consideration was given to the knowledge, attitudes, and beliefs of the target population (largely white, middle class, suburban). Consequently, the intervention was crippled from the beginning. Objectives were based on untested assumptions that mothers were not taking precautions that could prevent injuries to their preschool children in the home. Unfortunately, this assumption was never validated by a needs assessment of the young mothers' knowledge, attitudes, and practices. Thus, the program could never move beyond general content to specific practices that might have been amenable to change.

Also in contrast with Cases 1 and 2 was the use of the singular method of a twenty-minute discussion between a research assistant and a parent, followed by one phone call. It is not surprising that this limited intervention yielded limited results, as was demonstrated in the evaluation. As you will recall, the probability of a behavioral outcome is dependent on the frequency of learning opportunities and their rated effectiveness. Further contributing to the weakness of Case 3 was the fact that, although a complex evaluation design was used, seemingly none of the resulting information was fed back into redesigning the program. Instead, the program was labeled unsuccessful and apparently was discarded.

Organization and Conduct of Programs

The third essential competency of a health educator is the ability to organize and conduct the planned intervention. This involves changing the setting (first-order macro change) in order to explore and improve existing learning opportunities or to create new ones. Such change calls for developing a structure of organization, manpower, finance, and accountability for the purpose of shifting existing program processes. It may also include the assignment of new program responsibilities to newly created organizations. Table 9.3 shows how these variables were addressed for each of our three cases.

The sites where learning opportunities occur is a critical variable in the success of the intervention for a variety of reasons. First, if a site is not accessible to learners, obviously there can be no learning opportunity. Alternatively, if a site is unacceptable to the learner, little or no learning will occur. In Case 1, learning opportunities occurred in a number of different sites, including homes, hospitals, clinics, neighborhoods, community agencies, and legislative offices. This diversity of sites increased awareness of the problem for the total community and provided reinforcement of specific behaviors (the need for parents to supervise children, or obtain window guards). Case 2 also used a range of sites in providing learning opportunities. Initially, workshops were held in training centers; later, emphasis was shifted to schools, homes, shopping centers, and fairs. Unlike Cases 1 and 2, Case 3 used the clinic as the sole site for its learning opportunities. Given this limited site, the intervention in Case 3 was necessarily less likely to create change.

How programs are organized and the extent to which they are integrated into the existing functions of their sponsoring agency or organization are also critical elements of implementation. Integration is significant because health education programs are generally complex and cut across several functions of an organization. Failure to integrate an educational intervention has a direct relationship to the frequency of learning opportunities and their rated effectiveness. Case 1, for example, was a highly integrated program that was organized to involve the functions of public health nursing, housing inspection, outreach, and public information. This organizational structure, albeit complex, provided a much higher and more effective number of learning opportunities than might have been provided by a single health education program unit. Case 2, a program with a medium level of integration, functioned as a program of the Bureau of Maternal and Child Health and did not cut across other functions of

Table 9.3 *Organization and Conduct of Programs* (Cases 1, 2, and 3)

	Case 1	Case 2	Case 3
A. Site	Home, community agencies, hospital/clinic, neighborhood legal offices	Schools, playgrounds, training center	Clinic, home (phone call)
B. Organization	Integrated into public health dept. administrative functions	N.Y. State Dept. of Health Bureau of Maternal and Child Health	Prepaid medical plan special project
C. Personnel	Variety of public health workers, neighborhood volunteers, outreach persons, voluntary agency employees	State health dept. personnel, playground personnel, teachers, "consumer deputies"	Research assistant
D. Finance	Supported by the Office of Professional and Public Health Education, N.Y. City Dept. of Health	Contract with U.S. Product Safety Commission	Emergency Medical Services Research Grant, National Center for Health Services Research
E. Accountability	Citizens of N.Y. City through city health dept.	Citizens of N.Y. State and the U.S. Consumer Product Safety Commission through N.Y. State Dept. of Health	Members of prepaid Health Plan, National Center for Health Services Research

the department. However, there was a high degree of integration with the organizations where the problem occurred (schools, parks, recreation areas). Case 3 is an example of a program with little or no integration. Although well organized, it provided for no interaction with other parts of the prepaid clinic or the community.

Because people must be engaged as educators to conduct learning opportunities, personnel is a key variable in implementing health education. The competency of the educators and the acceptability of the educators to the learners are important issues. Case 1, with its complex organization, involved a variety of educators, with the health education specialist playing the coordinating role of "teacher's teacher." Staff development was encouraged to improve the competencies of other personnel in order to ensure a high-quality learning opportunity for learners. By using a large number of educators, the program made possible specialization by task and increased the likelihood that an educator would be acceptable to a learner (i.e., outreach workers indigenous to the community were used in counseling parents). Volunteers were used extensively in this program. It is widely known that volunteers are likely to be highly motivated, gregarious people—traits that assure their acceptance within the community.

In a similar manner, Case 2 utilized a range of personnel, including playground directors, recreation leaders, teachers, and "consumer deputies." Drawing from these community resources assured almost automatic acceptance within the community. To monitor competence, all participants were trained to conduct surveys of health hazards. In Case 3, however, the issues of the competence or acceptability of the research assistant/educator were not addressed.

How a health education program is financed is a fourth variable critical to its successful implementation. If a program is supported by the existing setting that desires change, it is likely to be continued. Alternatively, if a program is paid for through grants or contracts with other agencies or settings, continued funding is less likely to occur, because of the need to satisfy an agency that may have other interests competing for its financial resources. The program in Case 1 was financed by a city health department, using existing resources. In contrast, Cases 2 and 3 were supported by grants and contracts. Case 2 was paid for through a contract with the U.S. Product Safety Commission to the New York State Department of Health. Case 3 was supported by an Emergency Medical Services Research grant from the National Center for Health Services Research.

The final variable, accountability, is significant to implementation because every program must have processes of accountability built into them. By accountability, what we mean is that a program must be "valued" by decision makers and constituency groups. Generally, programs that are responsive to the needs of constituency groups and decision makers develop adequate mechanisms of accountability. Those programs that possess poor mechanisms of accountability tend to be discarded by decision makers on the grounds that they are not responsive to, and thus not supported by, their constituencies.

The program in Case 1 was accountable to the citizens of New York City through the City Health Department. Because it was supported by local funds, the program was monitored closely by administrators, politicians, citizens, and providers. To survive, the program had to develop ways to explain its purpose, objectives, and methods, and its significance to these constituencies.

Alternatively, Case 2 was accountable to the U.S. Consumer Product Safety Commission and to the citizens of the state of New York through a contract with the New York State Department of Health. The nature of the contract required that performance standards be met. Beyond meeting these requirements, however, the program provided for no other mechanisms of accountability that would assure its continued support, regardless of its success in creating change.

Similarly, Case 3 was accountable to the National Center for Health Services Research and the citizens of the United States through a federal Emergency Medical Services Research Grant. Although guidelines are placed on the expenditure of federal funds through grants, there are usually no other conditions specified. Thus, the researchers could select a setting, develop a program, and implement and evaluate it without needing to involve large numbers of consumers, providers, or other potential constituency groups. In such a program, because there is only indirect accountability to the public and no mechanisms for their involvement in the project, the public is placed at a distance, and real accountability is all but impossible to achieve.

Evaluation of Programs

The fourth essential competency of a health educator is the ability to evaluate educational interventions that are specific to a setting. As we discussed in Chapter 8, an evaluation has four fundamental aspects: (1) determining the social purpose of the evaluation, (2) determining the goals of the program, (3) developing criteria for measurement, and (4) selecting a research design for the evaluation. Table 9.4 (see p. 194) presents an analysis of our three cases regarding these aspects.

The social purpose of an evaluation is concerned with the question of why an evaluation is necessary. Defining the social purpose involves an examination of who wants the evaluation done and why. Depending on how these questions are answered, an evaluation may take varied shapes and proceed in different directions. In each of our three cases, the social purpose of the evaluation was to document the effect of a health educa-

Table 9.4 *Evaluation of Programs* (Cases 1, 2, and 3)

	Case 1	Case 2	Case 3
A. Social purpose	To save children's lives from window falls; to reduce financial burden of hospitalization, rehabilitation and maintenance	To reduce playground injuries and equipment hazards	To reduce injuries to children
B. Goals of program	1. To install window guards in tenements in high risk areas	1. To promote recognition of hazards for playground by recreation leaders	1. Parent recognition of hazards in the household
	2. To promote recognition of hazards of unguarded windows among population	2. To reduce hazards of playgrounds	2. Reduction of hazards in the household
		3. To reduce playground injuries	
C. Criteria for measurement	1. Number of window falls	1. To change participants' knowledge about playground hazards	1. Number of observed hazards in house
	2. Number of window fall fatalities	2. To reduce hazards on playgrounds	2. To change mothers' knowledge of household hazards
	3. Number of window falls after guards were installed	3. To reduce playground injuries	
D. Design of evaluation	Comparison of demographic data before and after intervention	Pre-test, post-test only (O-X-O design)	Post-test only; control group design (X-O design)

tion program upon a problem. Each case, however, had different constituencies to satisfy. Consequently, they focused on different dimensions of the problem.

The first two cases were concerned with the development of programs that would effectively create change. Case 1 focused on "saving lives" and, in so doing, was process oriented; the process created an awareness within the community and therefore increased the participation of a broad range of constituencies. Within this context, evaluation was continuous, occurring at various stages of the pilot program and later during the operational program. Case 2 emphasized environmental changes in the safety features of playground equipment. The implication was that these changes would reduce playground injuries to children. Based on this approach, the evaluation was concerned with measuring reductions in hazardous equipment rather than reductions in numbers of injuries.

Case 3 differed from the other cases in that its social purpose was to examine the effect of a given health education method designed to create change. The crucial difference, however, was that program development was not an important part of the social purpose, as it had been in Cases 1 and 2. Basically, the program in Case 3 was research oriented; a considerable amount of its resources was spent to develop an appropriate evaluation design. As a result, evaluation became the focal point of the program at the risk of minimizing the method.

In all three cases, the goals of the program were similar: each sought to reduce childhood injuries and fatalities. But because each program emphasized different dimensions of childhood safety, different methods were employed. These methods then determined the criteria that were used to measure goal attainment.

Case 1 was unusual because its criteria for measurement consisted of a discrete event that was readily observed and easily documented. The number of falls from windows and those resulting in fatalities were measured. The most powerful measure used was the number of falls from windows after guards were installed; this clearly documented the effect of the method. Although the program did not directly measure community participation, there was strong evidence that this participation occurred. The passage of a law could not have taken place without extensive documentation of the problem and community support for a specific method.

The criteria for measurement used in Cases 2 and 3 were alike. The reduction of environmental hazards was measured, along with changes in knowledge and attitudes. Evaluators thus measured the reduction in childhood injuries indirectly. Both cases shared the problem of not being able to link specific injuries or fatalities to their methods of intervention, as was possible in Case 1.

In each case the design of the evaluation emerged from the social purpose of the evaluation. Cases 1 and 2 emphasized program development as their purpose, in contrast to Case 3, which stressed research about a given method. Because of its social purpose, Case 3 developed an elaborate evaluation design that controlled for the effect of the method. Cases 1 and 2 used simple evaluation designs to document data before and after intervention. In Case 2 both pre-tests and post-tests were used to evaluate the effects of the program.

Involvement of People

The fifth and final essential competency of a health educator is the degree to which the health educator involves people in the totality of the change processes. In Table 9.5 we have analyzed, for our three cases, the degree to which people were involved in the total process from assessment of the setting through evaluation of the project. In setting up Table 9.5 we have referred to the involvement of people as the degree to which the community was involved in each case. We looked specifically at the involvement of (1) consumers, (2) direct service providers, (3) other providers, (4) community groups, and (5) decision makers.

Our examination in Chapter 8 of change in communities provides us with some valuable insights that will enhance our understanding of the role of community involvement in a community health education project. In Chapter 8 we distinguished between process goals and task goals: process goals are oriented toward the capacity of the community to function over time, whereas task goals are concerned with delimited functional problems in the system. In Chapter 8 we also described three types of community interventions: locality development, social planning, and social action. Locality development refers to a community's capacity to engage in cooperative problem solving on a self-help basis and to use processes of participative membership and participative decision making as part of the change process. The social-planning approach is oriented toward the solution of specific problems and is hierarchically organized, with planning and policy personnel as the decision makers. The social-action approach is generally concerned with empowering community members so that they can act as informed and effective change agents with the aim of changing the system.

Case 1 dealt with both task and process goals. The task goal was to reduce injuries to children resulting from window falls. The process goal involved community members in the process of acting as community educators. By involving large numbers of community members and community agencies as active participants in the task, the program enhanced the committment to the community by both the consumers who live in the area and the providers who work there. This last point refers especially to the high involvement of direct service providers—the police, hospital personnel, etc. The inclusion of indirect providers to help with the process of problem solving provided a bridge between neighborhood communities

Table 9.5 *Involvement of People* (Cases 1, 2, and 3)

	Case 1	Case 2	Case 3
A. Consumers	Locality-development, community-organization approach: high-level involvement	Social-planning approach: medium-level involvement using specified groups	Social-planning approach: no involvement
B. Direct service providers	Police, fire dept., hospital and public health, nurses, outreach personnel	Playground directors, supervisors	None
C. Other providers	Media experts, public and private agencies	Schoolteachers, nurses, PTA groups	None
D. The community	Community-based groups, community school boards, PTA's, supermarket chains, churches, block associations, tenant groups	Volunteers from consumers groups and women's groups	None
E. Decision makers	Legislators, community leaders, community groups	Playground directors, project directors	None

and the larger community, New York City. The development of this bridge proved effective in enlarging the number of individuals engaged in community participation and identifying themselves as community members. The inclusion of neighborhood community groups (churches, tenant groups) represented a community organization effort to determine that participation in the program was shared by a major segment of the community. The case description is unclear in specifying who were the actual decision makers. Coordination was supplied by the city health department, but it is probable that neighborhood community groups had their own participative decision-making organization, while agency and business enterprises had hierarchical decision-making structures. In spite of this mixed bag of decision makers, the community members collaborated to complete the task. The final test of the effectiveness of community involvement and collaboration was the passage by the city legislature of a law mandating window guards.

Case 2 is primarily task oriented: playground injuries were to be reduced and playground hazards eliminated. The social-planning approach was used; a problem was discovered, and a plan to eliminate the problem was prepared and implemented. Specific consumer groups were involved, including unpaid volunteers from local PTA's and consumer groups. The plan called for playground supervisors and volunteers to assess hazards and for playground directors to eliminate hazards. The participation of community members in the project was restricted to direct providers and to "consumer deputies" who functioned as indirect providers. The decision makers were the playground directors (who assumed the responsibility to reduce hazards) and the director of the project. The social-planning approach did accomplish the designated tasks, but with minimal community involvement and with little attention to furthering community process goals.

Case 3 was also representative of the social-planning approach. The goal was to reduce injuries to children in the home. The plan called for an educational intervention by a single individual and the design of a sophisticated evaluation. Mothers who were members of the Columbia Medical Plan were the target group. Consumers were involved only as passive recipients of the intervention and were not asked to actively participate. No effort was made to engage the participation of direct or indirect providers. There was no community involvement and also no attempt to involve community members in decision making related to the subject. It would seem that a major reason for the failure of Case 3 in achieving its goal was the failure of the plan to include the active participation of community members in the process.

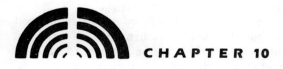

CHAPTER 10

Roles, Activities, and Functions of the Health Educator: Past, Present, and Future

This book began with a statement of the challenge to health care in the present decade—a challenge brought about by the second public health revolution, which has led to a need to rethink theory and method for influencing health behaviors in a pluralistic society. We have, in response to that challenge, provided a theory of change and an operational definition of health education as a method of change involving an understanding of settings, outcomes, and skills as they affect health education practice. We have compared and contrasted three cases of health education practice in order to illustrate how health educators create change. Our final task is to provide, within the context of the previous chapters, a description of the roles, activities, and functions of health educators. Because we believe in the value of a historical perspective for understanding this material, we have divided our discussion into three sections: past roles, activities, and functions; present activities and functions; and future directions.

Past Roles, Activities, and Functions

The emergence of the role of public health educator began in the United States in the first half of the nineteenth century. Responding to increased public interest about the care of the human body and the com-

199

mon health problems of the day, these first health educators functioned
primarily as journalists and public speakers rather than as teachers.
Throughout the nineteenth and the first half of the twentieth centuries,
their principal activities consisted of lecturing and preparing pamphlets,
newsletters, news releases, films, and exhibits. Many health administrators
during this period advocated popular education as a method of prevention
for the purpose of effectively reducing the high incidence of communicable
diseases, high infant and maternal mortality rates, and poor sanitation.

The dissemination of information was based on the belief that knowledge about health problems would result in better health practices. Early
in the twentieth century, small groups of individuals who were engaged in
health education practice began to believe that knowledge of the facts
alone neither assured people's motivations to change nor achieved the
goal of improving health practice. Their convictions led to a shift in the
philosophy of health education: instead of limiting the role of the health
educator to that of publicist, the new educational philosophy stressed an
active educational function that involved learners in the learning process.
The health practitioners who embraced this new role came largely from
backgrounds in teaching rather than journalism and public relations.
Functioning as educators, they began to develop learning experiences for
others that were directly related to health and to work directly with
people in face-to-face settings.

By the 1930's, community organization had become a major function
of public health educators. Mayhew Derryberry, Chief of Health Education Services in the U.S. Public Health Service from 1942 to 1963, was a
major sponsor of this new idea. Community organization remained the
dominant theme of health education from the 1940's through the 1960's.
The influence of this method and the high repute in which it was held, are
clearly shown by the public health legislation of the period—notably the
enacted legislation that required consumer organization and participation
in the "Great Society" programs for urban renewal, model cities, and
neighborhood health centers. Another example was the requirement that
the Peace Corps use the community organization method of "learning
through participation" as a principal approach in developing countries.

Bowman (1976) has summarized thirteen studies concerned with the
functions of public health educators (see Table 10.1, pp. 202–207). The
summaries include the methodology used in obtaining each study, the participants studied, and the principal findings about the activities, functions,
and roles of public health educators. Bowman warns us, however, that the
principal findings reported in these studies should be examined with the
understanding that they lack both common objectives and selected participants from different populations. He cautions the reader that because of
these differences and differences in methodology, the findings should be
compared in only the most general terms.

The thirteen studies can be examined in terms of their three principal methodologies: job analyses, time studies, and role perceptions. The studies cover the period from 1955 to 1970. Looking at the job-analysis studies, for example, we can see a trend away from the dissemination of information and preparation of informational materials. We can note a further trend in the movement of health educators away from the community organization activities of the 1950s and toward an emphasis on the behavioral approach and on training, program planning, and evaluation. The time studies, which are concerned with specific functions or activities of public health educators, also reveal that the amount of time spent by health educators on information dissemination has decreased since the 1950's. The three studies that used role perceptions as a principal methodology, which were carried out in the 1960s, further support the trends noted in the job-analyses and time studies: specifically, the perception of the role of the health educator as a planner and evaluator.

Present Roles, Activities, and Functions

By the 1960's and 1970's, public health educators began turning away from the community organization model in an effort to respond to new directions in health care, concerning the delivery of health services, that were brought about by the national legislation of that period. This new approach was and is referred to as the behavioral approach. The swing away from the concepts of participative membership, participative learning, and work with the community as the unit of change, to a statement of behavioral objectives with focus on individual behavior change was evidenced in the 1960's in a report of the Society of Public Health Education (SOPHE). The report gives special attention to determinants of human behavior, application of concepts of human behavior in program planning, program development, and program evaluation. The application of research findings to health education practice was also emphasized.

Evidence of the continued popularity of the behavioral approach, with its strong emphasis on behavioral objectives and planning, can be seen in the publication of Lawrence Green et al. (1980). In 1979 Green was director of the Office of Health Information and Health Promotion (OHIHP), a national bureau created in 1976 by Public Law 94-317 that speaks on national policy for health education. Community health education, however, continues as a viable approach and is well represented by the recently founded International Journal of Community Health Education (1978), edited by George Cernada.

The national health legislation enacted toward the end of the 1960's and in the early 1970's created many new programs that both expanded health services and made them accessible to larger numbers of people. It

Table 10.1 *Summary of Studies Concerned with the Activities, Functions, and Roles of Public Health Educators in the U.S., 1947 to Present*

Study	Methodology	Participants Studied	Principal Findings on Activities, Functions, and Roles
Rash, 1949	Job analysis through interviews using check list of duties and rating scale for estimates of time distribution	75 health educators from 7 midwestern states including 26 employed by health agencies	Health educators employed in health agencies devoted time to 46 different duties with greatest amounts spent on activities concerned with administration, education, and public relations.
Derderian, 1952	Job analysis employing checklist of functions, questionnaire, personal interviews	46 health educators employed by official and voluntary health agencies in Massachusetts	Activities reported by a high percentage of health educators were letter writing (85%), attending meetings (76%), distributing pamphlets (70%), writing and editing annual reports (61%), distributing posters (59%), writing reports (56%), giving consultant service (56%), attending staff meetings (51%). School health, program evaluation, research on methods and materials, and coordination of existing programs were most neglected activities.
Milne and associates, 1953	Time study	Health educators in state and local health departments in Mississippi	46% of time spent in school health activities; 12% in sanitation activities; 6 to 7% each in activities concerned with tuberculosis, acute communicable diseases, and maternal health.
Bureau of Health Education, California State Department of Public Health, 1954	Time study through use of self-coding report form	Health educators and other professional staff employed by the Bureau	Greatest portion of time spent in consultation and field services to local communities and health agencies; next largest blocks of time claimed by preparation of materials, administration and supervision, and professional development.

Anderson, 1954	Time study and examination of agency annual reports	Health educators in 38 local health departments in U.S.	50% of time devoted to dissemination of health information, publicity, and public relations; 20% to technical assistance and consultative services; 15% to community organizations, groups, and health projects; 10% to administration; and 5% to promotion and improvement of health education and inservice training.
Galiher and Wright, 1955	Job analysis employing personal interviews	Random sample of 171 (11%) members of APHA Public Health Education Section	Activities taking most time were working with professional groups, writing, organizing lay groups, planning meetings, and supervision of other staff; those taking least time were research, layout and printing, budget, information service, teaching, fund raising, and speaking. Activities considered to be most important were organizing lay groups, working with professional groups, planning meetings, and writing; less important were speaking, layout and printing, teaching, fund raising, information service, and research.
Bowman, 1957	Time study through use of self-coding report form to determine activities, and questionnaire to analyze frequency of duties and responsibilities assigned or requested	100 health educators graduated from schools of public health between 1943 and 1952 and employed by state and local official agencies in 33 states and 4 territories in U.S.	Over 25% of time was spent on activities concerned with communication or dissemination of information; 22% on health education programs, school health and staff education and training; 17% on administration; 15% on consultant functions; 6% on professional development; 6% on public relations; 5% on community organization and service. In contrast, duties requested of them most frequently related to public relations followed by consultation, communication or dissemination of information, community organization and service, administration and education.

Continued

Table 10.1 *Summary of Studies Concerned with the Activities, Functions, and Roles of Public Health Educators in the U.S., 1947 to Present (Continued)*

Study	Methodology	Participants Studied	Principal Findings on Activities, Functions, and Roles
Arnold, 1962	Questionnaire to determine perceptions of roles of public health educators, physicians, and public health nurses	40 teams in 23 local health departments in California selected on a modified random basis; each team consisted of 1 public health educator, 1 physician, and 1 public health nurse	Agreement on 35 of 58 listed activities; 14 of 35 activities attributed to health educators. Public health educators perceived as liaison public relations experts between health departments and outside agencies and as workers to carry and extend health department programs to public; giving service outside the agency; as coordinators of training within the health department; *not* perceived by selves or by physicians or nurses to be responsible for activities in program planning and evaluation to extent physicians and nurses were.
Delgado-Murphy, 1962	Questionnaire and interviews to determine perceptions of role of public health educators; time estimates of health education activities	38 public health educators employed at local or territorial levels in Puerto Rico plus 350 coworkers in these health agencies and related organizations	27 roles were enumerated by educators; when 14 of these were scrutinized quantitatively and qualitatively the 9 ranked as outstanding were: planner, guide, team member, resource person, instructor, coordinator, leader, organizer, interpreter of the profession. Highest percentage of time spent in program planning and evaluation followed by serving as health education resource, community organization, inservice education, preparation and use of education materials.
Danielsen de Lugo, 1966	Time study to determine activities	94 health educators employed at local and regional levels in Puerto Rico.	52% of work time devoted to specific functions with organization of medical services, personnel training, and preparation of materials claiming the most time followed by administration, collaboration in general

Author/Year	Method	Sample	Findings
			agency activities, and transportation; only 12% of this work time was used in working with clients and community groups and leaders with the remaining 40% used in working with personnel on training, consultation, program planning and evaluation within the agency.
Wang, 1968	Questionnaire to determine perceptions of the role of the public health educator including analysis of tasks performed most frequently	245 health educators graduated from schools of public health and employed in local, official, and voluntary health agencies in U.S.	Increase noted in role as program planner and evaluator, supervisor, administrator, trainer, community organizer and promoter of health education activities, and extension of health education through communication; decreased role in mass media and public relations. Noted need for more preparation for these and in education and training methods, consultation, psychology of learning and group methods, and research methods in health education.
Bowman, Bowman, and Roccella, 1969	Time study through use of self-coding report form to determine activities	90 health educators graduated from schools of public health between 1957 and 1966 and employed by local, state, or regional official agencies widely dispersed in U.S.	About 23% of time was spent on activities concerned with administration; 22% on health education programs, school health, and staff education; 18% on communication or dissemination of information; 13% on consultant functions; 7% on community organization and service; 6% on public relations; 6% on professional development; 3% on research and studies. Breakdown of items within these activities compared with the 1957 study above, more time was devoted to joint planning of health education programs, community organization, and person-to-person communication; less time was devoted to school health activities, mass media communication, and serving as resource on educational methods and media.

Continued

Table 10.1 *Summary of Studies Concerned with the Activities, Functions, and Roles of Public Health Educators in the U.S., 1947 to Present (Continued)*

Study	Methodology	Participants Studied	Principal Findings on Activities, Functions, and Roles
Bowman and O'Rourke, 1970	Job analysis employing questionnaire to assess involvement of public health educators in functions specified by SOPHE statement	98 health educators graduated from schools of public health since 1957 and employed in local, state, or regional official agencies widely dispersed in U.S.	Health educators consistently felt more qualified when involved in the 63 selected activities, the difference being statistically significant. Activities in which they were most involved and qualified were those related to community analysis to establish needs and set educational objectives followed by (in rank order) leadership in developing educational aspects of programs; formulating educational goals and policies; implementation of educational components of programs; staff leadership for development of health education activities, methods, and materials; community organization and coordination with groups and agencies including schools; administration, supervision, and recruitment; publication of reports and program experiences; staff education, training, and professional development; identification of needed educational research and study problems. Specific activities for which they felt well-qualified and least involved were those in school health, recruitment and training of health educators, continuing and staff education, and health education research.

| Bureau of Health Education, California State Department of Public Health, 1970 | Job analysis employing survey interviews to assess Department needs for health education services | Chiefs, assistant chiefs, and administrative officers of all 7 Department programs and the 24 elements or units within these programs. | 30 of the 31 program elements indicated need for health communications and health information services, 28 for training services, 27 for services in planning and evaluating education activities, 25 for community organization services, and 25 for consultation services. 23 of the 31 elements named all 5 areas of function as needed to reach program objectives in the next 2 fiscal years. |

Source: Reprinted from Robert A. Bowman, "Changes in the Activities, Functions, and Roles of Public Health Educators," *Health Education Monographs* 4, no. 3 (Fall 1976): 232–36; copyright 1976 by the Society for Public Health Education.

was a period of many changes. Most important among these were lifestyle changes, the rise of the ecology movement, increased concern for the effects of smoking and substance abuse, awareness of the problem of adolescent pregnancy, concern for patient and human rights, and a recognition of the need for increased accountability of health professionals and health programs. These changes have had a major impact on both the practice and education of health educators.

Health educators are now employed in a number of new settings, initiated in the 1970's. Health educators in the area of patient education, for example, practice in both hospital and clinic settings, as well as in outreach and follow-up programs for patients. A major new function of health educators, both in traditional and nontraditional health agencies, is training allied health personnel in methods applicable to changing health-related behavior. These allied personnel include nurses, teachers, and numerous other groups, such as personnel from child care agencies or rural cooperative extension programs. Unions and management now employ health educators to focus on problems of occupational health. Health maintenance organizations have become major employers of health educators in order to develop and implement preventive programs both in physical and mental health. This is only a partial list of emerging settings and of the new roles and activities that health educators are being called upon to perform. There can be no doubt that the area of health education has continued to expand since the studies we have cited in this chapter were completed.

The fact that the number of possibilities for health educators to practice is now far greater than at any time in history has important implications for the profession. First, there are problems for the colleges and universities that engage in pre-service and in-service education for practitioners. Should undergraduate and graduate curricula be revised to reflect the emergence of new settings for practice, new skills required by changes in roles and functions of health educators, and the increasingly prominent role health educators are being asked to assume as evaluators and researchers of the outcomes created by their activities? Should in-service education be broadened and expanded to provide practitioners with a necessary updating of their past knowledge and skills? Second, there is the problem of defining our profession in terms of its mission and its role with respect to other professions. Should health education develop a professional identity that can be translated through licensing requirements and standards of practice into laws that certify practitioners and offer legislative protection to those who have met minimum educational and experience qualifications? We will return to this question later in the chapter.

We have seen the major function of health educators change from dissemination of information to community planning and, now, to a behavioral emphasis. It would seem that the roles and functions of health educators and the settings in which they work are largely determined by social forces. *Healthy People* (1979), the recent Surgeon General's Report that we have mentioned in earlier chapters, seems to reflect a current mode of thinking in the field of health. Affirming that the next public health revolution must address the prevention of disease (namely, cardiovascular disease, cancer, and death and disabilities due to accidents), the report states that we must address our careless habits, our careless misuse of the environment, and the fact that we continue to permit harmful social conditions to exist. Thus, health educators, as a reflection of both national policy and social forces, are currently being asked to focus on interventions that will change individual lifestyles. Too great an emphasis on an individual's responsibility to control his or her life while minimizing the effect of socioeconomic forces, however, can place an undue burden on a large segment of society. Usually it is the better off and better educated who have both the means and the opportunity to acquire a safer car, a more nutritious diet, a medical checkup, and regular exercise. The disadvantaged members of society are too poor to make these expensive choices and frequently too burdened with work and worry to give extra thought, time, and money to do what is involved. William Ryan (1970) warns of an even greater mistake if we emphasize individual change while failing to attend to the effect of social forces on health. He describes this emphasis as a "brilliant ideology for justifying a perverse form of social action designed to change, not society as one might expect, but society's victim."

Future Directions: The Outlook for Health Education in the 1980's

What is the outlook for the practice of health education in the 1980's? Specifically, will health educators continue to define themselves as change agents? Will we be able to define the roles and activities of health educators sufficiently to insure their uniform preparation and adequate standards of performance? What will be the arena of practice of health education?

A recent publication of SOPHE and the Association for the Advancement of Health Education, *Health Education of the Public in the 80's* (1981), speaks of a "new wave" of health promotion and prevention. Four initial sets of assumptions are associated with this "new wave" of effort to expand the health delivery system (as expressed by Simmons and Nelson in the above publication):

1. The major determinants of health are lifestyle, environment, human biology, and medical care.

2. A key role of the health care delivery system is to prevent illness

(through lifestyle and environmental changes) and to identify risk
factors and disease early in their course.

3. The health care delivery system cannot work efficiently unless patients know when to use and when not to use, the system, and are
skilled in using specific procedures related to self-care.

4. Clinical, intervention will not succeed without patients' full cooperation in planning and carrying out therapeutic regimens.

The "new wave" is threatened, however, by the undertow of cost containment. This leads to a fifth assumption, one that reflects contractions of
health services:

5. All interventions implemented by the health care delivery system
ought to be cost effective.

How has health education, caught in this struggle between expansion
and contraction, responded to this new set of assumptions? We will look
at the responses of six major areas of the health care system: primary care
practice, health maintenance organizations (HMO's), hospitals, schools,
industry, and community settings.

Health Education in Primary Care Practices

Simmons and Nelson (1981) have described some models of primary
care practice that emphasize the role of health education. The following
four models are representative of the range of practices currently being
developed.

1. *Donald Catino, M.D., New London, New Hampshire. Solo Internal
   Medicine Practice. Targets: Chronic Disease, Weight Loss.* The physician in this solo practice has become increasingly interested in incor-
   porating health education concepts into the care rendered to all
   patients, no matter what the chief complaint. However, he has developed a special interest in helping his patients lose weight through a
   systematic educational program that has been developed. Elements
   of the program include a protein-sparing diet, individual counseling,
   behavior modification, guided use of self-help books on weight loss,
   and continuing care and reinforcement. About two hundred patients
   have begun the program, more than 70 percent of whom are still
   actively involved; the average weight loss has exceeded 25 pounds.

2. *Milton H. Seifert, M.D., and Associates, Excelsior, Minnesota. Small
   Family Medicine Group Practice. Targets: Patient Activation, Psychosocial Problems.* This small group practice is unique in several aspects.
   It is based on the premise that the "patient is properly the instructor
   of the provider." Taking cues from patients, the practice has responded in many concrete ways, such as: (a) hiring new personnel—
   a health educator (education background) and a living problems
   counselor (psychology)—to advance health education; and (b) organizing a Patient Advisory Council to provide continuous and legiti-

mate consumer input into the practice's decision making. Patient "problem limits" are negotiated between provider and patient, and a new language is being developed to describe patient problems in less pejorative terms or more descriptive language (e.g., reality disturbance versus hypochondriasis). The practice believes the greatest unmet health need is in the psychosocial area. Data from the practice indicate it is 4.5 times more likely to report mental and emotional problems than the National Ambulatory Medical Care Survey.

3. *Palo Alto Clinic, Palo Alto, California. Large Multi-Specialty Group Practice. Targets: Impairments, Diseases, Lifestyle Changes.* This large, multi-specialty group practice uses a centralized nurse-educator strategy for patient education. Patients are referred by their physician (via an "educational prescription") to patient educators, mostly former nurses, based in an "education center." The educators primarily rely on pre-packaged, mixed-media educational materials like those produced by Core Communications. The educational packages include patient pre-testing, use of videotapes, and take-home written materials, individual counseling, and patient post-tests.

4. *Wellness Resource Center, Mill Valley, California. Small Wellness Practice. Targets: "Wellness" through Nutrition, Physical Exercise, Relaxation-Medication, and Biofeedback.* The Wellness Resource Center (WRC) does not provide traditional medical care. Instead it emphasizes reaching for positive health. Clients go through a three-step process: (1) evaluation of health status, (2) education regarding new health behaviors, and (3) growth-trying new health behaviors. The "evaluation" phase uses mostly standard questionnaires to assess stress, physical tension, clinical symptoms, nutritional practices, and psychological outlook. The emphasis is on self-responsibility and self-knowledge through relaxation, communication, visualization, and creativity exercises (pp. 9–10).

Health Education in Health Maintenance Organizations

Health maintenance organizations (HMO's) are large-scale components of the health delivery system whose activities are similar to the primary well-being center referred to in Chapter 3. Mullen and Zapka (1981) have outlined their educational functions, which include (1) member orientation and relations, (2) patient and family education, (3) member health education and outreach to the community and to worksites, and (4) organizational development and in-service education.

The objective of member orientation and education is to promote optimal use of services, to encourage the use of services by high-risk members, and to develop member participation in the decision-making bodies of the HMO. Some of the aims of patient and family education are to increase adherence to therapeutic regimens, to provide patients and their families with a greater understanding of medical procedures, and to decrease the

stress of hospital and medical procedures. Educational guidance also has
the objective of reducing risk behaviors, for example, overeating and alcoholism.

The objectives of member health education and outreach programs include member education to manage minor ailments and to promote health
behavior (exercise, parent-child communication, and assertiveness training). Worksite programs represent another application of health education
outreach. These programs generally include stress management, physical
fitness and exercise, weight control and nutrition, control of alcohol,
smoking cessation, and hypertension control. Additional programs, to
provide in-service training and to improve HMO functioning, are designed
to sensitize providers to the various lifestyles and cultural styles of members and to improve staff satisfaction. These programs grow out of an
awareness that insensitive providers and poor working conditions can
have a negative effect on the health of members as well as staff.

An example of a health maintenance organization that has made the
effective use of health education is the Puget Sound Group Health Cooperative, one of the oldest HMO's in the country. Its comprehensive educational program consists of four major components: (1) consumer
orientation, (2) preventive care, (3) weight reduction and smoking cessation, and (4) the development of a consumer bill of rights.

Health Education in the Hospital Setting

Hospital-based patient education represents the area of greatest growth
in the use of health education in the final decade of the 1970's. Lee (1979)
provides us with the data to illustrate this growth; she found that the
number of hospitals with a patient education coordinating department increased from 1,218 in 1975 to 2,009 in 1978. After reviewing the American Hospital Association survey results, Lee concluded that "providing
patient education is regarded as a routine aspect of clinical practice for
clinicians, such as nurses, dieticians, and pharmacists hired by hospitals to
deliver patient care" (p. 11).

The typical model for the delivery of health education in hospitals involves the use of nursing personnel in programs that tend to focus on
inpatients and use informal bedside teaching, or on outpatients and use
formal, structured class sessions for patients who have specific diagnoses
or who share a common condition. A more comprehensive model of
health education, however, has been developed by Bernheimer and Ad-
cock (1979).

The Bernheimer-Adcock model is process oriented. It focuses on the
coordination of the multidisciplinary team that is responsible for the direct provision of the patient's basic medical care. The model brings together the treatment team to share their perspectives on the patient's
educational needs and the patient's readiness to respond to an educational

intervention. The process identifies which member (or members) of the team is most appropriate to deliver what aspect of the education at what particular time. The model provides for systematic feedback and coordination among the team of members, and concentrates on the functions of health education program planning, implementation, and evaluation in a free-standing office of health education.

Simmons and Nelson (1981), after examining the significant new health education developments now occurring in primary care settings, HMO's, and hospitals, have identified three major roles for health educators that have emerged from these settings. The two roles they have identified for those who work in primary care organizations are health education practitioner and health education consultant. As Simmons and Nelson explain these roles, "The practitioner is on the primary care facility staff and provides educational services for patients with special educational needs," whereas "the consultant works with the health staff in identifying educational problems and opportunities" and in "developing intervention strategies," including "methods to monitor and assess" the health staff's effectiveness and "to evaluate the benefits of the educational interventions." Health education consultants also "assist in the preparation of the health staff to carry out their respective educational roles." Simmons and Nelson note further that "in the process of developing the education-interventions," consultants "may engage in direct patient assessment" and in "the testing of procedures" and the "demonstration of methods." Thus, "in addition to the practitioner skills, the consultant should understand organizational behavior, problem analysis, have core management skills (e.g., program planning, management and budgeting), and have evaluation research expertise" (p. 15).

For complex organizations, such as hospitals and health organizations, Simmons and Nelson identify a third, administrative, health education role: the health education coordinator. Coordinators are responsible for "(1) setting priorities among potential educational activities; (2) catalyzing, planning, implementing, and evaluating individual educational programs; (3) budgeting; and (4) liaison with other departments and groups within the organization (e.g., medical staff, administration, nursing, discharge planning, etc.). The job is extremely difficult even under favorable conditions. Consequently, the skills required are similar in kind—though perhaps not as in-depth—to those needed by the consultant." Skiff (1977) also points out that the role of coordinator is not an entry-level position but one that represents a career advancement for an individual who has had other health work experiences.

Health Education in the Schools

Newman (1981), in assessing the school setting for health education, makes clear that the difficulties and challenges faced by education in the decade of the eighties will determine the direction of school health education. He lists the following factors as ongoing trends that will surely affect the future of health education, since they will have a significant impact on the development of education.

1. The status of teachers will continue to decline before the teaching profession can reestablish its credibility and nurture the renewed community support it needs to be effective.
2. Increased community pressure, best illustrated in declining financial support, will force a reduction in the breadth of educational activities offered by schools.
3. Teacher-training institutions and their programs will come under increasing scrutiny as they attempt to respond to public concerns about the quality of their graduates and, at the same time, suggest the need for longer (five-year) teaching degree programs.
4. Demands that teacher certification include some type of examination will increase, along with resistance to such a change from within teachers' organizations.
5. Accountability demands will increase further, fueling a renewed dialogue on the role of schools in our society.
6. Declining school enrollment in many areas and limited budgets will lead to requirements that more teachers be competent or certified to teach in more than one discipline area.
7. While supporting the 'back to basics' philosophy, the public will continue to demand that schools address such issues as drug and alcohol abuse, while avoiding such controversial topics as abortion. Planning bodies, like health system agencies, will focus attention on schools as they attempt to implement plans to improve community health status.
8. Stimulus for educational change from the federal government will decline so state education agencies and local school boards will have an opportunity to revert to old easy ways or to actively explore local initiatives to improve their individual systems (p. 33).

This list provides us with a somewhat pessimistic view of support for public education in the immediate future. We believe that this view can, however, be balanced by the continuing need for health education as a major topic in the public school curriculum. *The General Mills Family Report* (1979) provides us with a generalized needs assessment:

1. One-third or more of the parents questioned would be interested in participating in programs to help them (a) teach their children about sex (34%), (b) convince their youngsters not to smoke (37%), (c) deal with drug use among youngsters (49%), (d) feed their children nutritiously (32%), and (e) help their children cope with other health problems (34%).
2. There is a tendency for parents to deny health problems until they occur—this in spite of the fact that people, in general, are more con-

cerned about health and prevention than they were five years ago.
3. Seventy-five percent of American family members believe they are in good shape as long as nothing bothers them physically, and 54% don't even want to think about the fact that serious illnesses could happen to them or their friends.
4. Only 28% of adult family members feel well informed about health; only 24% feel well informed about nutrition; only 19% feel well informed about preventive medicine.
5. Women consider themselves better informed than men, and upper socioeconomic groups consider themselves better informed than lower socioeconomic groups.
6. Among those who considered themselves to be poorly informed about health, more than half were judged to be complacent in their attitude toward health.

If school health education is to prosper in the decade to come, several crucial areas must be addressed. Specifically, according to Newman, educators must (1) establish a clear foundation for health education planning, (2) articulate a clear focus for curriculum development and reimplementation, (3) expand the base for support of programs, and (4) rethink and reemphasize the concept of a school health team. The first area of activity addresses the need for goals and objectives. The second area focuses on method; the third, on the use of available resources. The fourth area raises the issue, Who is the school health educator?

Since our focus in this chapter is on roles and activities of health educators, this final issue requires some further discussion. All too often, health classes are taught by teachers whose principal training and interest are in other areas of the curriculum. The school nurse or health aide, on the other hand, is frequently the manager of the sick room and little else. The result is inadequate teaching and loss of student interest. The obvious solution would be to have a staff of trained health teachers and trained nurse practitioners. Anything short of this would compromise quality and make the idea of the school health team an empty concept.

Newman believes that the public's perceived need for further health education in the school will act as the force to create a dialogue between educators and the community on these four major issues. If this dialogue continues to develop and if it moves school health workers and community members closer to a consensus on these issues, then we may expect progress to continue and school health education to remain healthy in the period to come.

Occupational Health Education

We have previously defined occupational health in terms of health hazards and safety issues. Exposure to environmental hazards in the workplace threatens workers' health; in our earlier example from Chapter 4

workers exposed to piecework procedures in the garment industry were at
risk for carpal tunnel syndrome. The failure to provide and apply appropriate safety precautions also threatens workers' health. Occupational
health education includes educational activities to improve and preserve
the health of workers. Health education is the purview of many professionals in the work setting: physicians, nurses, safety engineers, industrial
hygienists, toxicologists, benefits representatives, exercise physiologists,
dieticians, and, last, health educators.

Have we prepared health educators to function in the industrial setting?
As Ware (1981) explains, the industrial environment offers some unique
challenges:

> Even the language is different. Perhaps most startling is the expectation
> that what the health educator undertakes will produce results in the
> direction desired by the company. Why have a program on promoting
> a beneficial health practice if the people do not change their behavior?
> Surely the voluntary smoking program you offer should cause a pro-
> portion of people to quit. There is no question that you, the health
> educator, can produce results. Likewise, it is taken for granted that you
> know what to do and how to do it, and what results your efforts will
> yield. Exhilarating as it is to be treated as the fully qualified profes-
> sional you are, the responsibility for success in terms of what the com-
> pany wants and expects can be a source of much frustration.

Nevertheless, Ware is cautiously optimistic. "The prospectus for health
educators in occupational health, whether in an industrial setting or in a
hospital," she believes, "at the least seems promising."

> The professional health educator has a unique composite of skills and
> knowledge that are not currently found in one person in occupational
> health. There's a need for the 'basics': a good scientific background in
> health and disease, in use of media, in designing training programs, and
> in teaching. For those health educators for whom advocacy and social
> action is a way of life, the constraints of most industries will be unbear-
> able. You might be more comfortable working for a union or for a
> government; yet these settings have their own constraints and priorities
> (p. 51).

Health Education in Community Settings

The focus of community health education in the eighties is on the individual, the goal is to educate the public toward a "medically proper lifestyle." Those health educators who perceive the community as a setting
where people can be taught to change to better health-related behaviors
cite information on the readiness of the American public to accept this
kind of learning. For example, a recent Louis Harris survey reports that
92.5 percent of those polled agreed that "if Americans lived healthier

lives, ate more nutritious food, smoked less, maintained our proper weight, and exercised regularly, it would do more to improve our health than anything doctors and medicine could do for us" (p. 57).

A model for community health education in the present decade is the Stanford University Heart Disease Prevention Program, a two-year experiment in three small California communities that was designed to determine whether an educational campaign could reduce the risk of cardiovascular disease. In the design of this study, two communities, Gilroy and Watsonville, were exposed to the educational intervention; the third, Tracy, was the control group. The results were encouraging. The overall risk of cardiovascular disease increased about 7 percent in Tracy over a two-year period. In Watsonville, however, the risk decreased 15 percent, and in Gilroy, the risk decreased 20 percent.

Despite the fact that the results of this project are encouraging, several problems, however, remain. First, the costs of community education programs of this kind are very high. Second, we do not know if the changes in behavior and lifestyle that have been reported will be maintained. Third, significant obstacles lie in the way of success in this kind of an approach, among them (1) the existence of community-based threats to health, such as poverty, racial discrimination, slum housing, and crime, obstacles over which individuals have little if any control; (2) the self-indulgent American lifestyle that is supported by a huge media industry and backed by much of the American corporate structure; (3) the inability of many people to accept the correlation between an indulgent lifestyle in the present and a disability in the future; (4) a health empire whose spokespersons tell us that we should put our efforts and money into high-technology cures; and (5) national policies that pay lip service to the aims of prevention, but, for example, subsidize tobacco growers.

How can health educators overcome these obstacles? If the direction of health education in the eighties is limited to a focus on changing one behavior, such as poor nutrition, to another (good nutrition), we will have only limited success. As Brown and Margo (1978) explain, "By focusing on behavior itself, health educators do not deal with the social relations and structures that may underlie and contribute to the behavior patterns they find objectionable and to the diseases they wish to prevent. The alienation of people from stressful working conditions, and inadequate nutrition due to insufficient income or inadequate food supply, are ignored." "The ultimate absurdity of this position," Brown and Margo continue, "is represented by a study of lead poisoning among children in Cleveland's black ghettoes. By focusing blame for the children's lead-paint eating on Southern blacks' permissive socialization of oral behavior, the researchers took the heat off the slumlords." Instead of focusing so intently on behavior, "community health educators must concern themselves in the present decade with the question: can community health educators develop a role in which they can help change the conditions that make people sick? We believe they can if they perceive their role primarily as advocate-facilitators for the constituencies that need their help" (p. 9).

The Future of Health Education as a Profession

Having described the various roles and activities of health educators in the major settings in which they currently function, we now ask, What is the future of health education as a profession? In order to answer this question, it is necessary to clearly define the specific competencies of health education specialists and the educational preparation that they require.

Foremost among the problems in defining the profession is the diversity of preparatory programs. Henderson *et al.* (1981) report that health educators are prepared in 108 bachelor, 83 master, and 31 doctoral-level programs. These programs are found in schools of public health, schools and colleges of education and health and of physical education and recreation, and other divisions of institutions of higher learning. There is no single set of accreditation standards for this diversity of programs and, therefore, no single set of guidelines to define their curriculum. This lack of specific standards for preparation has led to some confusion among employers, consumers, and third-party payers.

What competencies should the health education specialist have? What assurance do we have that education services are of high quality? Which health education services should be reimbursable by either national or private health insurance? Three forms of credentialing have been suggested as solutions to these problems. These include (1) accreditation of educational programs, (2) certification of personnel by the profession itself, and (3) licensure by a government agency.

The first phase of this effort toward credentialing and setting of standards began in 1978 when the Bureau of Health Professions and Health Resources Administration (Department of Health, Education, and Welfare) sponsored a conference of forty health educators from across the country. This group explored the similarities and differences in the preparation and practice of health educators in school, community, and medical care settings. The second phase of this effort was the forming of a project for a role-delineation study of health education. The first step of this work was completed in January 1980. The basic professional skills of entry-level health education practitioners were identified (this level was tentatively set at the completion of the bachelors degree), and seven major areas of responsibility of entry-level practitioners were enumerated.

These are (1) communicating health and health education needs, concerns, and resources; (2) determining the appropriate focus for health education; (3) planning health education programs; (4) evaluating health education; (5) coordinating health education activities; and (6) acting as a resource for health information and health education.

Figure 10.1 (see p. 220) diagrams the relationship between the role-delineation and credentialing processes. It is hoped that the Role Delineation Project and the subsequent movement by health educators toward credentialing will solve the problems created by the diversity of preparatory programs and result in acceptable standards for both preparation and practice in the profession. If this task can be accomplished in the decade of the eighties, the profession of health education will have come of age.

The Role of Colleges and Universities in Professional Preparation

Winder (1982) interviewed program chairpersons of two major graduate programs in California, one at UCLA and the other at the University of California, Berkeley. They were asked their perceptions of the direction of health education graduate training in the coming decade. The program chairpersons at both universities recognize the diversity of practice and the need for their institutions of higher education to provide some leadership. They have participated in a first step in this direction by creating a substantive dialogue in health education between West Coast schools. The Consortium for Health Education and Research of the Pacific (CHERP) has begun to meet and make this dialogue a reality, and the establishment of a blue-ribbon committee on a state level to plot strategies to improve health education in both the public and the private sectors has been discussed by the members.

In spite of this seeming progress, however, Winder, summing up the results of his interviews, is "forced to the conclusion that both educational institutions seem to have retreated from health education's preoccupation with changes in the macro systems of society. The UCLA program description provided for an educational experience in this direction. The program itself, however, was primarily oriented toward behavioral science rather than health education. The program at Berkeley is primarily directed toward changing the health-related behavior of individuals with only a minor emphasis on changes in organizations and communities." It would appear, at least from the information obtained from these two prestigious training programs, that they both represent, through their educational practice, a retreat from the teaching of theory and skills that students need to practice community health education. We can only hope that their faculty will reassert their leadership roles and reverse this trend.

Figure 10.1 *The Relationship Between Role-Delineation and Credentialing Processes*

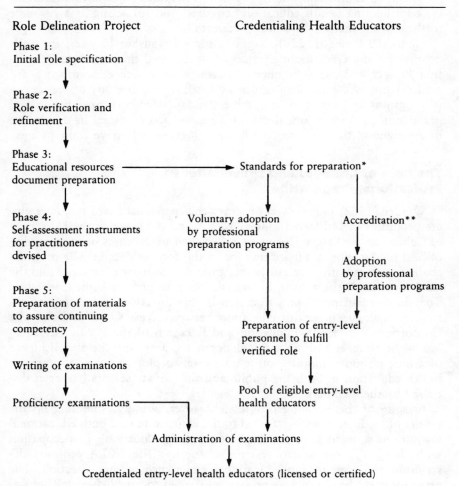

Role Delineation Project

Credentialing Health Educators

Phase 1:
Initial role specification

Phase 2:
Role verification and refinement

Phase 3:
Educational resources ⟶ Standards for preparation*
document preparation

Phase 4:
Self-assessment instruments for practitioners devised

Voluntary adoption by professional preparation programs

Accreditation**

Adoption by professional preparation programs

Phase 5:
Preparation of materials to assure continuing competency

Preparation of entry-level personnel to fulfill verified role

Writing of examinations

Pool of eligible entry-level health educators

Proficiency examinations ⟶

Administration of examinations

Credentialed entry-level health educators (licensed or certified)

Notes: *Endorsed by Association for the Advancement of Health Education; American College Health Association; American Public Health Association; American School Health Association; Society of Public Health Educators; Society of State Directors of Health, Physical Education, and Recreation; and Conference of State and Territorial Directors of Public Health Education.

**For example, by Council on Education, National Commission for Accreditation of Teacher Education for Public Health, North Central Association of Schools and Colleges, and state teacher credentialing authorities.

The Challenge of the 1980's

We can now turn our attention to the last question we raised in the introduction to this section, namely, What is the arena of health education in the eighties? We have surveyed health education practice in primary care facilities, hospitals, health maintenance organizations, schools, occupational health settings, and the community. Clearly, health education practice is marked by diversity. Just as clear, however, is an absence of programs that reflect second-order change. A strong swing toward the libertarian position on social values and the attendant undertow of cost containment policies that marked the opening years of the decade, strongly suggest a retreat from second-order change in the field of health care. We believe this trend will characterize health education practice for the coming decade.

Will health educators, then, continue to define themselves as change agents? Current practice reflects a commitment to first-order change in individuals, but not to second-order change, which involves change in organizations and communities. Indeed, Ware's admonition that health educators adapt to the norms and rules of corporate life if they wish to be effective runs counter to the whole concept of second-order change. If we define change in its broadest sense, we are witnessing health educators' retreat from a role that in earlier decades formed their professional identity.

Finally, the success of the Role Delineation Project suggests that the profession is working toward uniform guidelines for preparation and credentialing. But let us be forewarned: guidelines set at this time may freeze newly defined roles into practice at a moment in history that reflects health educators' activities in retreat from a more idealistic and egalitarian vision of their mission. We will, if this happens, find that Ryan's accusation, that we are pursuing a path of social action designed to change not society, but society's victim, applies to us.

Glossary

Access An individual's (or group's) ability to obtain health care. Because access has geographic, financial, social, ethnic, and psychic components, it is very difficult to define and measure operationally. Many government health programs have as their goal improving access to care for specific groups or equity of access in the whole population.

Accountability To be accountable means to furnish a justification or detailed explanation of financial activities or responsibilities; to furnish substantial reasons or convincing explanations. Accountability entails an obligation to periodically disclose, in adequate, detailed and consistent form to all directly and indirectly responsible or properly interested parties, the purposes, principles, procedures, relationships, results, incomes, and expenditures involved in any activity, enterprise, or assignment, so that they can be evaluated by interested parties.

Acute disease A disease that is characterized by a single episode of a fairly short duration from which the patient returns to his or her normal or previous state of health or level of activity. Although acute diseases are frequently distinguished from chronic diseases, there is no standard definition or distinction. For example, an acute episode of a chronic disease (e.g., an episode of diabetic coma in a patient with diabetes) is often treated as an acute disease.

At risk The state of being subject to the occurrence of some uncertain event that connotes loss or difficulty.

Behavior modification One major theory of learning, also referred to as the stimulus-response, associationist, or social-learning theory. Modification refers to changing an individual's response by stimulus substitution or altering the response by manipulating the environment.

Bimodial distribution A distribution of observations characterized by a number of observations clustering at two different points on the distribution.

Biomedical research Research concerned with human and animal biology, and with disease and its prevention, diagnosis, and treatment. It contrasts with "health services research," which is concerned with the organization, effects, and other aspects of health services.

Bureaucratic model Used to describe a type of relationship between a client and an intervenor, the bureaucratic model expresses a client-to-professional (i.e., qualified expert) relationship. In the exchange, the client surrenders responsibility to the intervenor for those actions that are necessary to change the client.

Categorical program Originally, a health program that concerns itself with research, education, control, and treatment of only one or a few specific diseases. More generally used for programs concerned with only a part, instead of all, of the population or health system.

Cause Something that, if prevented, removed, or eliminated, will prevent the occurrence of an event in question; and, if permitted, introduced, or maintained, will be followed by the event in question.

Chronic disease Disease that has one or more of the following characteristics: results in permanent residual disability; is caused by nonreversible, pathological alteration; requires special training of the patient for rehabilitation; or may be expected to require a long period of supervision, observation, or care.

Cognitive field theory One of two major theories used to explain how people learn human behavior. In this theory, learning occurs as "insights" or new meanings a person has acquired. Learning is identified with "thought" (cognition) and is purposive, explorative, innovative, and creative. Insights occur when individuals, pursuing their own purposes, see new ways of using the elements in their environment.

Collaborative model Used to describe a type of relationship between a client and an intervenor, this model implies partnership between the parties. The identification of the client's needs is a shared responsibility, and the intervention is jointly implemented by both client and intervenor.

Community organization A process by which a community identifies its needs and objectives, organizes into groups to work on identified problems, develops confidence and will to work together, takes action in respect to these problems, and in doing so, develops cooperative attitudes and practices within the community.

Conditioning Produces changes in a response habit and is achieved by stimulus substitution. Substitution is accomplished by accompanying an adequate stimulus with a new stimulus or by response strengthening or modification, which either strengthens the stimulus or changes it.

Consumer model Used to describe a type of relationship between client and an intervenor, this model describes the client as a consumer who enters the marketplace, seeking specific services from an intervenor (a change agent). The consumer purchases these services for a price negotiated between the two parties.

Criteria Predetermined measures against which access, continuity, efficiency, appropriateness, or quality of health education services may be compared. For example, criteria for appropriate patient education for a urinary tract infection may be specific knowledge of the importance of a urine culture. Criteria are often used synonymously with guidelines.

Dependent or independent variable An independent variable is a stimulus acting on the organism. A dependent variable is a response of the organism and usually occurs in the form of a behavior.

Diagnosis The art and science of determining the nature and cause of a disease and of differentiating among diseases.

Disease Previously considered to be a moral or legal problem, literally "without ease," disease is the failure of adaptive mechanisms of an organism to react adequately or appropriately to stimuli and stresses to which it is subjected. This maladaption results in a disturbance in the function or structure of some part of the organism. Disease to a large extent is socially defined; for example, drug dependence presently tends to be viewed as a disease, whereas it was previously considered to be a moral or legal problem.

Distribution curve A graphed curve that reflects the way observations distribute themselves. Usually the frequency of the observations are plotted along a vertical axis, and the observations themselves are plotted along the horizontal axis.

Effectiveness The degree to which diagnostic, preventive, therapeutic, or other action or actions achieves the intended result. Effectiveness requires a measurable outcome based on the action taken. It does not require consideration of the cost of the action, although one way of comparing the effectiveness of actions with the same or similar intended results is to compare the ratios of their effectiveness to their costs.

Efficiency The relationship between the quantity of inputs or resources used in the production of medical services and the quantity of outputs produced.

Epidemiological analysis A type of analysis based on a statistical association between a characteristic and a disease.

Epidemiologist A public health scientist whose interest is in the occurrence of disease by time, place, and persons.

Epidemiology The study of the distribution of a disease or a physiological condition in human populations and of the factors that influence their distribution.

Etiology The science of causes or origins of disease.

Evaluation A process of measuring the effects of a program against specific predetermined goals or outcomes as a means of contributing to subsequent decision making about the program and improving the future performance of the program.

Facility The place where health care is provided, used synonymously with site (e.g., buildings, including physical plant, equipment, and supplies). One major type of health resource, facilities include hospitals, nursing homes, and ambulatory care centers. The term has not been used to include the offices of individual practitioners.

First-order change Change from one behavior to another that occurs from within a group.

Gestalt field theory(ies) A process of learning in which learning is defined as gaining new insight, outlooks, or thought patterns. Gestalt theorists view individuals, their environments, and their interactions with their environments as occurring simultaneously, and define this as the "field."

Goal A quantified statement of a desired future state or condition (e.g., an infant mortality of less than twenty per thousand live births, a physician-to-population ratio greater than four per thousand, or an average access time for emergency medical services of less than 20 minutes).

Goal-attainment model of evaluation One of two major approaches to evaluation, this model views evaluation as a measure of the degree of success or failure encountered by a program. It uses program goals to measure outcomes.

Group dynamics The process of interaction of an individual and the group, group dynamics is concerned with the effect of a group upon an individual's readiness to change or to maintain certain standards or norms. According to Lewin, all psychological events (e.g., thinking, learning) are functions of mutual relationships. Together they define both person and environment in mutual interaction.

Group theory Originally proposed by Galois to describe a group (e.g., number, objects, concepts, events), group theory has been used by Watzlawick to explain change from within a group and change from outside a group.

Health belief model Used to explain health-related behavior in terms of belief patterns, this theoretical model includes as factors susceptibility, severity, costs, and benefits of treatment, and cues to action.

Health care delivery system An organized system of services, personnel, equipment, and facilities in which persons, families, groups, and communities receive services to prevent disease, and to diagnose and treat illnesses.

Health education (1) An operational definition: a deliberately planned, structured learning opportunity (or opportunities) about health that occurs in a setting at a given point in time and involves an interaction between an educator and a learner. (2) A process definition: a change in health-related behavior in individuals or groups that leads to an improvement in health status for those individuals or groups.

Health maintenance organization (HMO) An entity with four essential attributes, it is (1) an organized system for providing health care in a geographic area, for which the entity accepts the responsibility to provide or otherwise assure the delivery of (2) an agreed-upon set of basic and supplemental health maintenance and treatment services to (3) a voluntarily enrolled group of persons, (4) for which services the HMO is reimbursed through a predetermined, fixed, periodic prepayment made by or on behalf of each person or family unit enrolled in the HMO, without regard to the amount of actual services provided.

Health promotion Specific intervention strategies that occur at the primary level of prevention designed to (1) make the host stronger or more resistant to infection, (2) decrease the effect of the agent upon the host, and (3) create a barrier in the environment that prevents the agent from reaching the host.

Health services research Research concerned with the organization, financing, administration, effects, or other aspects of health services, rather than with human biology and disease and its prevention, diagnosis, and treatment. In a sense, health services research concerns itself with the form, and biomedical research with the content, of medicine.

Health status   A means of describing and measuring the state of an individual's health or the health of a population.

Holistic-inductive reasoning   A method of reasoning used mostly in the social sciences involving a process of thinking that moves from the specific to the general, from the part to the whole.

Homeostasis   The physiological mechanisms of the body that permit it to maintain a balance among internal physiological conditions such as temperature, sugar, air, and salt.

Homeostatic mechanisms   Responses developed by the body to achieve a stable state either for the whole organism or between different but interdependent body systems.

Humanistic medicine   Medical practice and culture that respects and incorporates the concepts that the patient is more than his or her disease and the professional is more than a scientifically trained mind using technical skills. Both are whole human beings interacting in the healing effort. People are more than their bodies. They are a unique, interdependent relationship of body, mind, emotions, culture, and spirit.

Hypothetico-deductive reasoning   A method of reasoning, used largely by natural scientists, that involves the use of assumptions in order to test out ideas logically or empirically (e.g., an experiment).

Iatrogenic   An illness resulting from actions taken by the healer to treat a disease (e.g., a drug reaction).

Illness   Although usually defined synonymously with "disease," there are important differences between the two terms. *Illness* is used to subjectively describe a negative state of health. It is present when an individual perceives himself or herself as diseased (i.e., having discomfort or "dis-ease"). *Disease* is the term used to objectively describe a state of negative health. It is present when identifiable by objective, external criteria.

Input measure   A measure of the quality of services based on the number, type, and quality of resources used in the production of the services. Health services are often evaluated by measuring the education and training level of the provider, the reputation or an accreditation of the institution, the number of health personnel involved, or the number of dollars spent, as proxy measures for the quality of the service.

Laboratory method   A type of experiential learning occurring within a community or group. New patterns of behavior are invented and tested in a climate supportive of change in behaviors.

Lifestyle(s)   Ways of behaving; refers to the sequence of physical, social, and mental experiences that make up the existence of the individual or group.

Locality development   One of three major approaches used to create change at the community level, locality development emphasizes process goals designed to improve the capacity of the community to engage in cooperative problem solving. Use of democratic method is of central importance.

Morbidity The number of persons in which a disease is present; usually expressed as a rate (e.g., the proportion of persons with disease to the total population).

Mortality The number of deaths that have occurred in a given time or place; usually expressed as a rate (e.g., the proportion of deaths to the total population).

Multiple causation The idea that a given disease has a number of different causes, which can be divided into three general categories: (1) host-related factors (factors linked to characteristics of the human population), (2) agent-related factors (factors associated with the specific cause), and (3) environmental factors (factors within the surroundings of both agent and host).

Needs assessment A process used by health educators to identify the needs of a target population, needs assessment includes working with the population to determine what needs to be changed and exploring alternative ways or methods to implement the changes.

Objective A quantified statement of a desired future state or condition with a stated deadline for achieving the objective (e.g., an average access time for emergency medical services of less than 30 minutes by 1985). The educational planning process specifies objectives that will, when implemented, achieve its goals.

Occupational health services Health services concerned with the physical, mental, and social well-being of people in relation to their work and working environment and with the adjustment of people to work and work to people.

Outcome measure A measure of the quality or effectiveness of health education in which the standard of judgment is the attainment of a specified end result or outcome.

Planning The conscious design of desired future states as described in a plan by its goals and objectives, planning incorporates the description of and selection among alternative means of achieving the goals and objectives, and the conduct of those activities necessary to the design (e.g., data gathering and analysis) and the activities necessary to assure that the plan is achieved.

Policy A course of action adopted and pursued by a government party, statesman, or other individual or organization; any course of action adopted as proper, advantageous, or expedient. Health educators rarely make policy. They may, however, have significant influence on policy formulation.

Policy formulation Keeping need, resources, demand, technological alternatives, and maximum participation in focus throughout the program-planning process so as to accomplish the kind of public education that will encourage policymakers to adopt the proposed program.

Practice The use of one's knowledge in a particular profession. The practice of health education is the exercise of one's knowledge and skills of educational theory in the promotion of health and treatment of imbalance among internal physiological conditions.

Primary prevention Specific interventions designed to reduce the outbreak (new cases or incidence) of disease in a population in a given time period. Usually these strategies include health promotion and specific protection.

Process goals Statements of direction or desire that are concerned with how something is accomplished rather than what or why it is accomplished. Process goals emphasize means rather than ends (e.g., a concern for interaction of people instead of the task at hand).

Psychosomatic illness The presence of bodily physical symptoms that result from mental conflict.

Quality The nature, kind, or character of someone or something; hence, the degree or grade of excellence possessed by the person or thing.

Refreezing A process of internalizing a new behavior by an individual, refreezing is the third phase of Lewin's process analysis of change or learning. Unless new attitudes are refrozen, individuals, organizations, or communities may easily return to earlier, more familiar behavior patterns.

Reliability In research, the reproducibility of an experimental result (i.e., how closely a repeat of the experiment would yield the same answer, whether or not correct).

Response modification If a response has already been conditioned to a stimulus, a new response can be conditioned to the original stimulus, thereby modifying the original response.

Risk assessment A technique of epidemiological analysis used to identify those specific subgroups within a population that have a higher risk or chance of acquiring a given disease.

Risk factors Factors known to be associated with an increasing risk of an individual acquiring a specific disease.

Salutogenesis The origin of health rather than disease.

Salutogenic model A model that locates an individual's position on the ease/disease continuum.

Secondary prevention Refers to specific interventions that attempt to reduce the presence of a previously existing disease (i.e., the prevalence of a disease) in a population. Secondary prevention strategies usually include screening, casefinding, diagnosis, and treatment of disease symptoms.

Second-order change Change from outside the group that results in movement of the group to a higher logical type (e.g., change from one way of behaving to another way of behaving).

Service A specific unit of health care provided to a population.

Social action One of three major approaches used to create change at the community level, social action emphasizes both task and process goals. Objectives usually entail the modification of policies of formal organizations (e.g., cause-specific activities of trade unions or welfare rights organizations).

Social-learning theory One of two major theories used to explain how people learn human behavior, social-learning theory is based on four principles—drive, cue, response, and reward—that form a learned response. A cue is a stimulus that sets off an internal response to satisfy a drive, and external behavior follows.

Social planning One of three approaches used to create change at the community level, social planning emphasizes the solution of substantive social problems (e.g., mental health departments, commissions on alcoholism).

Somatic Related to the body, as distinguished from the psychic or social.

Stimulus-response theory A learning theory stating that learning can be described as the response of an individual to a stimulus, generally from the external world.

System A way of thinking about a human problem. The elements of a system are an environment, inputs into the system, and outputs from the system.

Systems model A theory that looks at the world in terms of the interrelatedness and interdependence of all phenomena, and, within this framework, at a phenomenon as an integrated whole whose properties cannot be reduced to those of its parts. Living organisms, societies, and ecosystems are all systems. Living systems consist of subsystems that are wholes in regard to their parts, and parts with respect to the larger wholes.

Systems model of evaluation One of two major approaches to evaluation, the systems model views organizations as pursuing other functions besides the achievement of predetermined (ideal-state) goals. These functions include the acquisition of resources, coordination of subunits, and adaption of the organization to its environment. The model is concerned with measuring, not simply the achievement of goals themselves, but the ability of an organization to establish itself as a "social unit" that is capable of achieving a goal.

Task goals Statements of desired outcomes that emphasize concern for what is to be done and focus upon accomplishment of objectives.

Tertiary prevention Specific interventions used to assist diseased or disabled people in a population. Tertiary prevention strategies are directed toward reducing the impact of existing disabilities on the overall quality of peoples' lifes.

Theory of logical types Used by Watzlawick to explain change from outside the group, this theory involves a process by which a class (a set of group members) moves (i.e., changes) to a higher logical level. Watzlawick uses the phrase a "change of a change" to explain it.

Treatment The management and care of a patient for the purpose of combating disease or disorder.

Unfreezing The first phase of Lewin's three-part process of change. Learning occurs when an individual can make an informed choice of whether to change an already existing behavior. The learning, or change, process that leads to an informed choice is based on unfreezing previous attitudes, beliefs, and behaviors and creating a receptivity to new knowledge that may provide the basis for the development of new ideas. Once unfreezing has occurred, individuals are able to experiment with alternative attitudes and behaviors, which they may then adopt.

Validity   The degree to which data or results of a study are correct or true; the extent to which an observed situation reflects the true situation.

Voluntary health agency   Any nonprofit, nongovernmental agency, governed by lay or professional individuals (or both), organized on a national, state, or local basis, whose primary purpose is health related.

Web of causation   An illustration or map of those hypothesized relationships that are believed to exist between a problem (or disease) and the environmental, host, and agent factors that have caused the problem to appear.

Well-being center   A basic unit of the health care delivery system organized to provide people with learning opportunities about health. As defined by Blum, a well-being center would be a place where people learn about new health behaviors and issues that result in the ill health of populations, and organize themselves to solve health problems.

References

Antonovsky, A. 1979. *Health, Stress, and Coping.* San Francisco: Jossey-Bass.

Appley, D., and Winder, A. E. 1973. *Groups in A Changing Society: Introduction to T-Groups and Group Psychotherapy.* San Francisco: Jossey-Bass.

————, eds. 1977. "Collaboration in Work Settings." *Journal of Applied Behavioral Science* 13, no. 1.

Argyris, C. 1970. *Intervention Theory and Method: A Behavioral Science View.* Reading, Mass.: Addison-Wesley.

Bahnson, C. B. 1975. "Psychologic and Emotional Issues in Cancer: The Psychotherapeutic Care of the Cancer Patient." *Seminars in Oncology* 2: 293–308.

Becker, M., and Maiman, L. 1974. "Socio-behavioral Determinants of Compliance with Health and Medical Care Recommendations." *Medical Care* 13: 10–24.

Belloc, N. B., and Breslow, L. 1972. "Relationship of Physical Health Status and Health Practices." *Preventive Medicine,* 1:415–21.

Bennis, W. G. 1969. *Organization Development: Its Nature, Origins, and Prospects.* Reading, Mass.: Addison-Wesley.

Berkman, L. F. 1977. "Social Networks, Host Resistance, and Mortality: A Follow-up Study of Alameda County Residents." Ph.d. dissertation, Department of Epidemiology, School of Public Health, University of California, Berkeley.

Bernheimer, E. 1977. *Shared Leadership—A New Approach to Patient Care.* Atlanta: U.S. Public Health Service, Center for Disease Control, Bureau of Health Education, no. 47.

Bigge, M. L. 1964. *Learning Theories for Teachers.* New York: Harper and Row.

Biller, R. P. 1971. "Some Implications of Adaptation Capacity for Organizational and Political Development." In *Toward a New Public Administration,* ed. Frank Marini, p. 93. Scranton, Pa.: Chandler Publishing Company.

Blake, R. R., and Moulton, J. S. 1964. *The Managerial Grid.* Houston: Gulf Publishing.

————. 1976. *Consultation.* Reading, Mass.: Addison-Wesley.

Blockstein, W. L.; Bailey, A. R.; and Hansen, R. H. 1973. "Expanding the Role of a University in Consumer Health Education." *Health Education Monographs* 3: 62–69.

Blum, H. L. 1976. *Expanding Health Horizons: From a General Systems Concept of Health to a National Health Policy,* pp. 51–54. Oakland, Calif.: Third Party Associates.

———. 1978. "Does Health Planning Work Anywhere, and If So, Why?" *American Journal of Health Planning* 3, no. 3.

Boston Women's Health Collective. 1980. *The Boston Women's Health Book Collective International Women and Health Resource Guide.* West Sommerville, Mass.: Boston Women's Health Collective.

Bowman, R. A. 1976. "Changes in Activities, Functions, and Roles of Public Health Educators." *Health Education Monographs* 4: 226–46.

Bradford, L. P.; Gibb, J. R.; and Benne, K. D. 1964. *T-Group Theory and Laboratory Method.* New York: John Wiley and Sons.

Bronowski, J. 1973. *The Ascent of Man.* Boston: Little, Brown and Company.

Brown, E. R. and Margo, G. E. 1978. "Health Education: Can the Reformers Be Reformed?" *International Journal of Health Services* 8, no. 1.

Campbell, D. T. and Stanley, J. C. *Experimental and Quasi-Experimental Designs for Research.* 1973. Chicago: Rand McNally Publishing Company.

Cartwright, D. 1949. "Some Principles of Mass Persuasion: Selected Findings of Research on the Sale of United States War Bonds." *Human Relations* 2: 253–67.

Cassel, J. 1974. "Psychosocial Processes and Stress: Theoretical Formulation." *International Journal of Health Services* 4: 471–82.

Churchman, C. W. 1979. *The Systems Approach and Its Enemies.* New York: Basic Books.

Cochrane, A. L. 1972. *Effectiveness and Efficiency: Random Reflections on Health Services.* London: Nuffield Provincial Hospitals Trust.

Cox, T. 1979. *Stress.* Baltimore: University Park Press.

Derryberry, M., ed. 1952. "Expert Committee on Health Education of the Public." *World Health Organization Technical Report,* Series No. 89. Reprinted in *Focal Points* (Bureau of Health Education, Center for Disease Control), April 1980.

Dershewitz, R. A., and Williamson, J. W. 1977. "Prevention of Childhood Household Injuries: A Controlled Clinical Trial." *American Journal of Public Health* 67: 1148–53.

Dollard, J., and Miller, N. E. 1950. *Personality and Psychotherapy.* New York: McGraw-Hill Book Company.

Donabedian, A. 1973. *Aspects of Medical Care Administration: Specifying Requirements for Health Care.* Cambridge, Mass.: Harvard University Press.

Dubos, R. 1965. *Man Adapting.* New Haven: Yale University Press.

Dunn, W. N., and Swerczek, F. W. 1977. "Planned Organizational Change: Towards Grounded Theory." *Journal of Applied Behavioral Science* 13: 135–158.

Elinson, J., and Hear, C. E. A. 1970. "A Social Medical View of Neighborhood Health Centers." *Medical Care* 8: 97–103.

Engle, T. L. 1964. *Psychology: Its Principles and Applications.* 4th ed. New York: Harcourt, Brace and World.

Engle, T. L., and Schmale, A. H. 1972. "Conservation-Withdrawal: A Primary Regulatory Process for Organismic Homeostasis." In Ciba Foundation, *Physiology, Emotion, and Psychosomatic Illness* (Symposium 8). Amsterdam: Elsevier.

Etzioni, A. 1960. "Two Approaches to Organizational Analysis: Critique and Suggestion." *Administrative Science Quarterly* 5: 257–78.

Farquhar, J. 1972. "Community Approaches to the Study of Cardiovascular Disease." *American Journal of Epidemiology* 96: 36.

Feldman, J. J. 1966. *The Dissemination of Health Information.* Chicago: Aldine Publishing Company.

Fisher, L.; Goddard, V. H.; Quinn, J. V. B.; Alison, J.; and Maio, P. C. 1980. "Assessment of Pilot Child Playground Injury Prevention Project in New York State." *American Journal of Public Health* 70: 1000–1002.

Fox, J. P.; Hall, C. E.; and Elveback, L. R. 1970. *Epidemiology: Man and Disease,* pp. 83–88. New York: Macmillan Company.

Fuchs, V. R. 1974. "Health, Economics, and Social Choice." In *Who Shall Live?* New York: Basic Books.

General Mills, Inc. 1979. *The General Mills American Family Report, 1978–79: Family Health in an Era of Stress.* Minneapolis, Minn.: General Mills, Inc.

Glaser, E. M. 1977. "Facilitation of Knowledge Utilization by Institutions for Child Development." *Journal of Applied Behavioral Science* 13: 89–109.

Golembiewski, R. T. 1969. "Organizational Development in Public Agencies: Perspective on Theory and Practice." *Public Administration Review* 29: 367–78.

Goodstein, L. O. 1978. *Consulting with Human Service Systems.* Reading, Mass.: Addison-Wesley.

Gordon, J. E., and Ingalls, T. H. 1958. "Medical Ecology and Public Health." *American Journal of the Medical Sciences* 235: 337–59.

Gori, G. B., and Richter, B. J. 1978. "Macroeconomics of Disease Prevention in the United States." *Science* 200: 1124–30.

Green, L. W.; Kreuter, M. W.; Deeds, S. G.; and Partridge, K. B. 1980. *Health Education Planning: A Diagnostic Approach.* Palo Alto, Calif.: Mayfield Publishing Company.

Greenberg, B. G. 1977. "Evaluation of Social Programs." In *Readings in Evaluation Research,* ed. F. G. Caro, pp. 155–74. New York: Russell Sage Foundation.

Greiner, L. E. 1967. "Patterns of Organizational Change." *Harvard Business Review* 45: 119–28.

Haynes, R. B.; Taylor, D. W.; and Snow, J. C., *et al.* 1979. "Annotated and Indexed Bibliography on Compliance with Therapeutic and Preventive Regimens." In *Compliance in Health Care,* ed. Haynes, R. B.; Taylor, D. W.; and Sackett, D. L., pp. 337–423. Baltimore: Johns Hopkins University Press.

Hazlett, W. H. n.d. Letter to the editor. *Medical Opinion and Review.*

Healthy People: The Surgeon General's Report on Health Promotion and Disease Prevention. 1979. Department of Health, Education, and Welfare (Public Health Service), Publication no. 79-55071.

Henderson, A. C.; Wolle, J. M.; Cortese, P. A.; and McIntosh, D. V. 1981. "The Future of the Health Education Profession: Implications for Preparation and Practice." *Public Health Reports* 96, no. 6.

Henig, R. M. 1976. "East Kentucky's Answer: A Model for the Future." *The New Physician* (June 1976), pp. 24–27.

Hilleboe, H. E., and Schaefer, M. 1968. "Evaluation in Community Health: Relating Results to Goals." *Bulletin of the New York Academy of Medicine* 44, no. 2.

Hinkle, L. E., Jr., and Wolff, H. G. 1957. "Health and Social Environment: Experimental Investigations." In *Explorations in Social Psychiatry,* ed. A. Leighton *et al.* New York: Basic Books.

Holmes, H. B., and Peterson, S. R. 1981. "Rights Over One's Own Body: A Woman-Affirming Health Care Policy." *Human Rights Quarterly* 3, no. 2.

Hull, C. L. 1943. *Principles of Behavior.* New York: Appleton-Century-Crofts.

Hutchinson, G. B. 1960. "Evaluation of Prevention Services." *Journal of Chronic Diseases,* pp. 497–508.

Illich, I. 1976. *Medical Nemesis: The Expropriation of Health.* New York: Random House.

An Interim Guide for Health Education in a Health Care System. 1978. Rockville, Md.: Bureau of Community Health Services.

Jacobs, S., and Ostfeld, A. 1977. "An Epidemiological Review of the Mortality of Bereavement." *Psychosomatic Medicine* 39: 344–57.

James, G. "Evaluation in Public Health Practice." 1962. *American Journal of Public Health* 52: 1145–54.

Kiritz, S., and Moos, R. H. 1974. "Physiological Effects of the Social Environment." In *Health and the Social Environment,* ed. P. M. Insel and R. H. Moos. Lexington, Mass.: D. C. Heath.

Knowles, J. H. 1976. "The Responsibility of the Individual." *Daedalus* (Fall 1976), pp. 57–80.

Koehler, W. 1925. *The Mentality of Apes.* New York: Harcourt, Brace, and Company.

Lalonde, M. 1974. *A New Perspective on the Health of Canadians: A Working Document.* Ottawa: Government of Canada, Catalog No. H31-1374 (April 1974).

Laszlo, E. 1972. *The Systems View of the World.* New York: Braziller.

Lauzon, R. R. J. 1977. "An Epidemiological Approach to Health Promotion." *Canadian Journal of Public Health* 68, July–August 1977.

Leavell, H. R., and Clark, E. G. 1965. *Preventive Medicine for the Doctor in His Community.* New York: McGraw-Hill.

Lee, E. 1979. *Reimbursement Forum Proceedings.* American Hospital Association, Bureau of Health Education Project, October 25, 1979.

Leshan, L. 1978. *You Can Fight for Your Life: Emotional Factors in the Causation of Cancer.* New York: Harcourt Brace Jovanovich.

Lewin, K. 1953. "Studies in Group Decision." In *Group Dynamics,* ed. D. Cartwright and A. Zander. New York: Row, Peterson, and Company.

————. 1961. "Quasi-Stationary Social Equilibria and the Problem of Permanent Change." In *The Planning of Change,* ed. W. G. Bennis, D. D. Benne, and R. Chen. New York: Holt, Rinehart and Winston.

MacMahon, B. 1961. "Principles in the Evaluation of Community Mental Health Programs." *American Journal of Public Health* 51: 963–968.

Mico, P. R. 1978. "An Introduction to Policy for Health Educators." *Health Education Monographs* 6 (Supplement 1): 7–17.

Milo, N. 1976. "A Framework for Prevention: Changing Health-Damaging to Health-Generating Life Patterns." *American Journal of Public Health* 66, no. 5.

Minkler, M. 1980–81. "Citizen Participation in Health in the Republic of Cuba." *International Quarterly of Community Health Education* 1, no. 1.

Mullen, P. D., and Zapka, J. G. 1981. "Health Education and Promotion in HMOs: The Recent Evidence." *Health Education Quarterly* 8, no. 4.

National Center for Health Education. 1978. "Planning for Health Education in Our Communities" (mimeographed).

Navarro, V. 1976. "Social Class, Political Power, and the State: Their Implications in Medicine." *Social Science and Medicine* 10: 437–57.

Neill, A. S. 1960. *Summerhill: A Radical Approach to Childrearing.* New York: Hart Publishing Company.

Newman, I. M. 1981. "Agenda for the 80s: School Health Education." In *Health Education of the Public in the 80's*. New York: Metropolitan Life Insurance Company.

Nuckolls, K. B.; Cassel, J.; and Kaplan, B. H. 1972. "Psychosocial Assets, Life Crisis, and the Prognosis of Pregnancy." *American Journal of Epidemiology* 95: 431–41.

Nyswander, Dorothy. 1956. "Education for Health: Some Principles and Their Application." *California's Health* 14:9.

――――. 1980–81. "Public Health Education: Sources of Growth and Operational Philosophy." *International Quarterly of Community Health Education* 1, no. 1.

Parkes, C. M. 1971. "Psychosocial Transitions: A Field for Study." *Social Science and Medicine* 5: 101–15.

Patton, M. Q. 1978. *Utilization-Focused Research*. Beverly Hills, Calif.: Sage Publications, Inc.

――――. 1980. *Qualitative Evaluation Methods*. Beverly Hills, Calif.: Sage Publications, Inc.

Peterson, W. 1966. "On Some Meanings of Planning." *Journal of the American Institute of Planners* 32: 137.

Pfeiffer, W. J., and Jones, J. E. 1974. *A Handbook of Structured Experiences for Human Relations Training*. La Jolla, Calif.: University Associates.

"Report of the 1972–1973 Joint Committee on Health Education Terminology." 1973. *Health Education Monographs* 33: 63–70.

Rice, A. K. 1969. "Individual, Group, and Intergroup Processes." *Human Relations* 22: 565–84.

Ring, R. "Inside Track: Sex Ed Tools." *Valley Advocate* (Springfield, Mass.), July 1, 1981.

Roemer, M. I. 1971. "Evaluation of Health Service Programs and Levels of Measurement." *HSMHA Health Reports* 86: 839–48.

Ross, H. S., and Mico, P. R. 1980. *Theory and Practice in Health Education*. Palo Alto, Calif.: Mayfield Publishing Company.

Ross, M. G. 1955. *Community Organization: Theory and Principles*. New York: Harper and Brothers.

Rothman, J. 1968. "Three Models of Community Organization Practice, from National Conference on Social Welfare." In *Social Work Practice*. New York: Columbia University Press.

Schulberg, H. C. and Baker, F. 1968. "Program Evaluation Models and the Implementation of Research Findings." *American Journal of Public Health* 58: 1248–55.

Scriven, M. 1971. "Evaluating Educational Programs." In *Readings in Evaluation Research*, ed. F. G. Caro, pp. 49–52. New York: Russell Sage Foundation.

Sharpson, M. 1974–75. "Factors Determining the Health Situation in Developing Countries." World Bank Staff Working Paper (draft), Washington, D.C.

Simmons, J. J., and Nelson, E. C. 1981. "Health Education in Health Care." In *Health Education of the Public in the 80's*. New York: Metropolitan Life Insurance Company.

Skiff, A. 1977. "Guidelines for a Clinical Internship in Hospital-Based Health Education." Report, College of Medicine and Dentistry of New Jersey, Office of Consumer Education, Piscataway, N.J.

Skinner, B. F. 1948. *Walden Two*. New York: Macmillan.

――――. 1971. *Beyond Freedom and Dignity*. New York: Knopf.

Sliepcevich. E. M. 1975. "A Concept of Health Education Skills." Unpublished paper.

Society for Public Health Education, Inc., and Association for the Advancement of Health Education. 1981. *Health Education of the Public in the 80s.* New York: Metropolitan Life Insurance Company.

Somers, A. R. 1969. *Hospital Regulation: The Dilemma of Public Policy.* Princeton, N.J.: Princeton University Press.

――――. 1976. In *Preventive Medicine USA: Health Promotion and Consumer Health Education* (Task Force Report). New York: Prodist.

――――, ed. 1976. *Promoting Health: Consumer Education and National Policy.* Germantown, Md.: Aspen Systems Corporation, 1976.

Somers, A. R., and Somers, H. M. 1977. *Health and Health Care Policies in Perspective.* Germantown, Md.: Aspen Systems.

Spiegel, C. N., and Lindaman, F. C. 1977. "Children Can't Fly: A Program to Prevent Childhood Morbidity and Mortality from Window Falls." *American Journal of Public Health* 67: 1143–47.

Suchman, E. A. 1967. *Evaluative Research Principles and Practice in Public Service and Social Action Programs.* New York: Russell Sage Foundation.

Sullivan, D. 1973. "Model for Comprehensive, Systematic Program Development in Health Education." *Health Education Reports* 1: 4–5.

Susser, M. 1974. "Ethical Components in the Definition of Health." *International Journal of Health Services* 4: 539–48.

Syme, S. L., and Berkman, L. F. 1976. "Social Class, Susceptibility and Sickness." *American Journal of Epidemiology* 104: 1–8.

Szasz, T., and Hollender, M. H. 1956. "A Contribution to the Philosophy of Medicine: The Basic Models of the Doctor-Patient Relationship." *Archives of Internal Medicine* 97: 585–92.

Terris, M. 1975. "Approaches to an Epidemiology of Disease." *American Journal of Public Health* 65: 1037–45.

Thorner, P. M. 1972. "Health Program Evaluation in Relation to Health Programming." *HSMHA Health Reports* 86: 525–31.

"Toward a Policy on Health Education and Public Health." Policy statement adopted by the Governing Council of the American Public Health Association, November 2, 1977. Reprinted in *Focal Points*, 1978, Bureau of Health Education Center for Disease Control.

Ware, B. 1981. "A View of Occupational Health Education: Practice, Problems, Prospects." In *Health Education of the Public in the 80s*, New York: Metropolitan Life Insurance Company.

Watzlawick, P. 1974. *Change: Principles of Problem Formation and Problem Resolution,* New York: W. W. Norton and Company.

Weckwerth, V. E. 1970. *On Evaluation: A Tool or a Tyranny.* Systems Development Project No. 9-4(15), *Comment Series.* Minneapolis: University of Minnesota Press.

Weisbord, M. R. 1976a. "Why Organization Development Hasn't Worked (So Far) on Medical Centers." *Health Care Management Review* 1:17–28.

――――. 1976b. "Organizational Diagnosis: Six Places to Look for Trouble With or Without A Theory." *Organization and Group Studies* 1: 430–47.

Weiss, C. H. 1972. *Methods for Assessing Program Effectiveness.* Englewood Cliffs, N.J.: Prentice Hall.

Winder, A. E. 1981–82. "Typical Activities of Health Educators in Public and Private Settings in California." *International Quarterly of Community Health Education* 2, no. 2.

Winkelstein, W. 1972. "Epidemiological Considerations Underlying the Allocation of Health and Disease Care Resources." *International Journal of Epidemiology* 1: 69–74.

"What Is Health Education?" 1947. *American Journal of Public Health* 37, no. 6.

Wolf, S., and Goodell, H. 1968. *Harold G. Wolff's Stress and Disease*, 2d ed. Springfield, Ill.: Thomas.

World Health Organization Report Summary. 1975. In "Mortality and Morbidity Trends, 1969–1972." *WHO Chronicle*, August.

Author Index

Subject Index

Other Mayfield titles of interest to health educators:

CASE STUDIES IN HEALTH EDUCATION PRACTICE
by Helen Cleary et al.

Selected case studies illustrate various types of health education practice in schools, communities, medical care, worksites, and international settings. The case studies help to bridge the gap between the study of theory and its practical application and will help newly emerging health educators to become more knowledgeable about the realities they will face on the job.

EVALUATION OF HEALTH PROMOTION PROGRAMS
by Richard A. Windsor et al.

This text offers a comprehensive overview of and case material relating to the theory, principles, and methods used in the evaluation of health promotion and disease prevention programs.

THEORY AND PRACTICE OF HEALTH EDUCATION
by Helen S. Ross and Paul R. Mico

This text describes how the health educator helps to resolve health problems, and it presents numerous theories, programs, and examples to show how behavioral theory may be applied in various settings.

HEALTH EDUCATION PLANNING: A DIAGNOSTIC APPROACH
by Lawrence W. Green et al.

A pragmatic, tested framework—the PRECEDE model—is used to evaluate and apply principles of health education intervention to problems involving community health, patient education, and school health education. Included are exercises that deal with specific health promotion situations.

MANAGING HEALTH PROMOTION IN THE WORKPLACE
by Rebecca S. Parkinson and Associates

A committee of nine health professionals shows how to set up health promotion programs or upgrade existing ones. In addition to the guidelines, 12 background papers and examples of health programs in 17 corporations are included.

BASIC STATISTICS FOR THE HEALTH SCIENCES
by Jan W. Kuzma

Statistical concepts, principles, and methods are presented in an easily understood manner to students of medicine, nursing, public health, and the allied sciences. This class-tested book features information on computer usage in biostatistics and useful learning aids for students.

CONTEMPORARY BEHAVIORAL THERAPY
by Michael D. Spiegler

This book introduces behavior modification theory and techniques that are used to change habits, motivations, and lifestyle. Included are participation exercises, case studies, and procedures for applying behavioral change techniques.

USING COMPUTERS IN THE BEHAVIORAL SCIENCES
by Paul C. Cozby

Designed exclusively for students in the behavioral and social sciences, this brief text introduces the major uses and applications of computers in basic research design and data collection. An assessment of the major statistical packages is included.

For further information, please contact Karen Letendre, Product Manager.

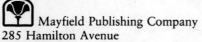 Mayfield Publishing Company
285 Hamilton Avenue
Palo Alto, CA 94301   (415) 326-1640